The path to emotional harmony with Bach flower remedies

A practical guide for everyday use

ZAKLINA ZIC

THE PATH TO EMOTIONAL HARMONY WITH BACH FLOWER REMEDIES

GRATITUDE

At the beginning of this book, I would like to say that I am infinitely grateful and happy to be able to help and relieve all those who have emotional problems, and there are too many of them in this world because it is simply the life we live. Life is an endless mix of emotions that we experience every day.

I am grateful to my sons Miloš and Vladimir, who have been my unreserved, constant support on the path of my personal and professional development. Thank you for believing in me and encouraging me in my work.

I am grateful to my brother Marjan, who has always been by my side throughout my life with his advice, support, and faith in me.

I am grateful to my mentor, Emira Antonić, who was always by my side and inspired me not to give up on my goal. Of course, I am grateful to everyone else who contributed in any way to the creation of this book.

Finally, I must say that even though my mother Ana is no longer with us and is a beautiful angel in heaven, I am grateful for all the sacrifices she has made for me over the years. And she always told me, "My dear, you are strong and smart, and I know you can achieve anything you set your mind to." I believe in you and the good deeds that you do for everyone around you. Thank you, mother, and I bow to your personality, huge heart, and kindness.

CONTENTS

AUTHOR'S MESSAGE

This book is for all those who want to achieve emotional balance in their lives. For all of you who want to achieve a sense of wholeness in your health, peace, and well-being, For all of you who want to achieve inner peace and balance with 100% natural solutions from the comfort of your home,

Are you tired of constantly fighting stress, anxiety, and emotional turmoil? Are you longing for a holistic and natural approach to restoring harmony to your life? Look no further! Dr. Bach's Flower Remedies are just what you need.

Unleash the healing properties of nature using the natural power of flowers. Dr. Bach's flower remedies offer a gentle yet effective way to achieve emotional well-being. From stress and anxiety to low self-esteem and a lack of focus, these flower remedies can help you find peace and harmony within yourself.

Begin your journey towards emotional balance! Explore the amazing world of Dr. Bach flower remedies and experience their amazing effects. Let these gentle yet powerful natural remedies bring you inner peace, harmony, and emotional calm. Embrace the power of nature and reclaim your emotional well-being today. I believe that in this book you will find yourself and everything you need to harmonise your life and the lives of your loved ones.

INTRODUCTION

Welcome to the world of Bach flower remedies, where the possibilities for healing and change open up before you. The book "The Path to Emotional Harmony with Bach Flower Remedies: A Practical Guide for Everyday Use" is your guide to discovering a unique treatment that provides complete harmony of mind, body, and spirit.

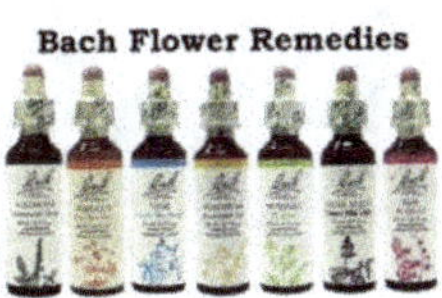

Bach flower remedies are delicate and powerful natural preparations made from plant extracts, designed by Dr. Edward Bach. His deep understanding of human nature led to the discovery of 38 different remedies, each with its own specific properties, that have the ability to help us deal with different emotional states. This book gives you a detailed insight into each individual's essence and how it can affect your emotional life. You get to know Dr. Bach's simple system of using remedies and how to use them in the most effective way. Learn how to recognise symptoms and emotional imbalances you may not notice and how to treat them using the right remedies. This book also offers numerous stories of individuals who have faced various challenges and found healing using Dr. Bach flower remedies. Their personal experiences can provide you with inspiration and hope that you too can achieve deep change and emotional balance in your life.

"The Path to Emotional Harmony with Bach Flower Remedies" is a comprehensive manual that will provide you with all the information and tools you need to achieve emotional well-being, release negative patterns, and find inner peace. Dive into the world of Bach flower remedies and discover the power of transformation that awaits you.

However, it is important to note that Bach Flower Remedies are not a substitute for professional medical advice, and for severe or chronic conditions, it is always recommended to consult with an authorised healthcare professional.

BACH FLOWER THERAPY: THE ORIGIN AND BENEFITS OF ITS APPLICATION

In the 1930s, the English physician Dr. Edward Bach created the principles of a new treatment system: treatment with 38 flower remedies. Treatment with Dr. Bach flower remedies gained real recognition after the Second World War, when it began to spread not only in Western Europe but also in America, Australia, India, etc. The ingredients of Bach flower therapy work on the body's energy system, and this treatment uses accumulated energy from flowers. With this method, there is no risk of overdosing or a wrong diagnosis (because then the drops will not help, but they will not hurt either).

The principle of treatment with this method is the old principle, "Heal yourself." In this sense, treatment with Bach flower remedies increasingly helps the professional treatment of psychosomatic diseases. With Bach flower therapy, the diagnosis is not based on physical symptoms but solely on the psychological and emotional state of the patient. As Dr. Bach says,

There is no true healing without peace of mind and an inner sense of purity!!!!!

Illness is based on the conflict between the soul and the spirit in body. Feelings of pride, hatred, anger, selfishness, greed, jealousy, envy, fear, and impatience are often the real causes of illness.

What is health? We often ask ourselves...

If a person behaves in complete harmony with his soul, he lives his life in complete harmony.

Each flower of Dr. Bach is the embodiment of a certain state of our soul. The human soul contains all 38 mental and spiritual states of flowers from Dr. Bach's system. Each person experiences Dr. Bach's flower remedies differently. The strength of a person's reaction depends on their degree of sensitivity as well as their willingness to change and take responsibility for their health.

How do I determine the combination of flower essences?

The key symptoms in the selection of flower remedies are the characteristic signs of blocked energy, for which the condition requires blooming energy.

It is very important that: you always treat what is happening in the present.

But they can also be treated:

a) Momentary feelings

b) Deeply rooted beliefs

c) Momentary shock

Bach therapy treats the person, not the disease; therefore, it is very important when determining the combination of Bach flower remedies to let the patient talk spontaneously about the problem he has and observe how the person expresses himself, the body's reaction, and the words he uses to express his feelings.

It is very important to find the right medicine.

The very attention we pay to the patient shows that we are there for him (this is the difference compared to allopathic medicine, which has no time for the patient himself).

The vibrations of the floral combination express strength through a person's emotions and help them become who they truly are.

Babies and animals respond very quickly to this therapy, unlike adults who think it's a placebo effect, because it works for them.

There are no contraindications for giving Bach flower therapy, which means that it can be used by small children, newborn babies, pregnant women, infirm people, etc. When a pregnant mother takes Dr. Bach's flower remedies, the baby absorbs only the vibration it needs. After birth, if the baby needs some flower essences, then the mother can take Bach drops if the baby is sucking, because that way the baby receives the vibration of the remedies. If a person is worried about the amount of alcohol in Bach flower remedies, the drops can be put in warm tea or milk where the alcohol evaporates or placed on the skin on the part of the hand where the pulse is felt, so that the information of the remedies passes to the baby's thoughts and emotions.

With Bach flower remedies, the vibrations of the essence penetrate our body and develop positive changes in us. By obtaining this motivation from the remedies, a natural balance is achieved in the organism. It may happen that two people with different characters need the same remedies because the medicine works individually, which is why the healing process can be slow or fast. The reason is that we, as personalities, immediately accept the beautiful and positive parts of our character, emotions, thoughts, and feelings, but when we need to accept those unpleasant, negative character traits, then it is more difficult, and it is precisely at this moment that the fantastic effect of Bach's flower remedies comes into play. Because they teach us to love the dark side of our personality, not just the lighter side. Parallel to the therapeutic combination of Bach flower remedies, rescue drops can also be used.

Bach flower remedies are not addictive; they do not change us but bring to the surface what we really are.

The only condition in which this therapy should not be administered is to alcoholics and drug addicts who are undergoing treatment and withdrawal and are using Antabuse therapy. In this case, they can use Bach flower remedies for external use, or when making drops, instead of 5–10 drops of alcohol, 5–10 drops of apple cider vinegar are placed in the therapeutic bottle.

The original package of Bach flower remedies contains 27% alcohol, and the rest is the vibration of the remedies.

The dosage of therapeutic Bach drops is at least 4 times a day for 4 drops in tea, milk, soup, water, etc. or directly in the mouth under the tongue, making sure that the pipette does not touch the tongue. Then keep the drops in your mouth for a few seconds, because that's where the greatest effect is. They can be dripped into a spoon and then drunk. It would be nice to take them more often, but it depends on the person himself and how much he is willing to fight for his health. The first dose of drops is taken immediately after waking up, the last in the evening before going to bed, and two or more times during the day. If a person uses it three times a day, the energy information from the flower will not be transferred, so it is very important to use it at least four times a day. There are no contraindications for taking the drops; they can be taken on an empty stomach, before meals, or after meals, so there are no rules; they are taken when it suits the person.

In cases of acute diseases or severe pain, it can be taken more often, e.g., 4 drops every 10–30 minutes until improvement. Bach flower drops can also be placed in a water bath or as a poultice (e.g., for sprains).

If used for transient moods, add 4 drops to tea, juice, or milk and drink sip by sip at intervals until you finish. When preparing a flower therapeutic bottle, you can combine the essences of a maximum of seven Bach flower remedies, which does not mean that there must be seven; sometimes 1-2 well-chosen Bach flower remedies are enough to defeat the disease.

If the remedy is taken regularly, the effect will not be absent, but if it is not taken regularly, it may have little or no effect. If the patient takes the remedies regularly and, after a while, starts to forget, it is a sign that the remedies have stopped working and a new consultation is needed.

With success, they are also given to pregnant women or women immediately after childbirth when depression appears due to too much responsibility or too many obligations.

The most important thing is to listen carefully to what the person has to say because it can be the remedy of mustard but also sweet chestnut. For example, if she is a single mother, she can fall into sweet chestnut depression.

This therapy is also given for nocturnal urination in children, but it is very important to find out what kind of attitude the parents have towards the children, whether the children have nightmares, maybe they want to attract attention (Chicory), or are jealous of their younger brother or sister (Holly or Star of Bethlehem). If the child is old enough, the problem should be discussed with the child, not with the mother.

The world has changed since 1936, but human nature has remained the same (for example, fear is the same today as it was in Dr. Bach's time). That is why Bach flower therapy is eternal.

However, it is important to note that Bach Flower Remedies are not a substitute for professional medical advice, and for severe or chronic conditions, it is always recommended to consult with an authorised healthcare professional.

GROUPING OF BACH FLOWER REMEDIES

Bach flower remedies are divided into 7 groups:

1. Fears

a) Rock rose

b) Mimulus

c) Chery plum

d) Aspen

e) Red chestnut

2. Uncertainty

a) Cerato

b) Scleranthus

c) Gentian

d) Gorse

e) Hornbeam

f) Wild oat

3. Disinterest

a) Clematis

b) Honeysuckle

c) Oliva

d) Wild rose

e) White chestnut

f) Mustard

g) Chestnut bud

4. Loneliness

a) Heather

b) Impatiens

c) Water violet

5. Too much concern for the people around you

a) Vine

b) Vervain

c) Beech

d) Chicory

e) Rock water

6. Too sensitive to the people around them

a) Holly

b) Centaury

c) Agrimony

d) Walnut

7.   Disappointment and hopelessness

a)   Larch

b)   Oak

c)   Crab apple

d)   Star of Betlehem

e)   Willow

f)   Elm

g)   Pine

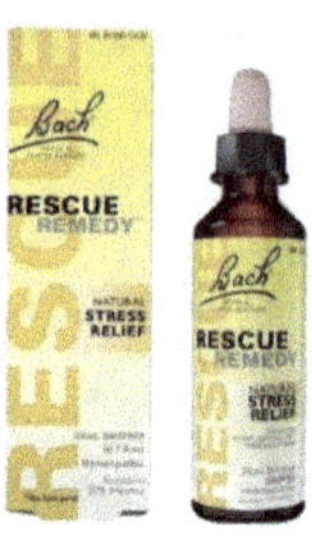

RESCUE REMEDY

Rescue drops, which are a combination of five flower remedies, are most often used. They are called emergency drops.

The flower remedies in the Rescue Drops system are:

1. Rock rose: for panic attacks and great fear

2. Star of Bethlehem: for a state of shock, shock here means any state that disrupts our energy stability, from the sudden sound of a knock on the door and hearing unpleasant news to physical injuries and loss of consciousness.

3. Impatiens: intolerance, irritability, violent and loud reactions to situations in life.

4. Cherry plum: great fear, hysteria; the person is afraid that he will lose control, that he will go crazy, and that he will do something terrible.

5. Clematis: during loss of consciousness or fainting, it helps a person to stand firmly on the ground and to return to himself. Rescue flower drops are used in cases of acute stress, when we have heard bad news, excessive worries before an interview, stress before a public performance, when we feel very nervous and tense, when we lose consciousness, in a state of shock, etc. These drops are a lifesaver until the arrival of medical help.

These drops are still prescribed:

• When a person is embarrassed by a family scandal or when he hears some unpleasant news;

• When a person works in stressful conditions, e.g., an emergency room, a slaughterhouse, etc;

• When we feel great fear, for example, when bitten by dogs, it is given to fathers who are waiting for their wives to give birth (then they are nervous and impatient);

• Mother and baby receive Rescue remedy and Oliva immediately after delivery due to exhaustion;

• Given to children when teeth are growing, it helps against pain. You can put drops on the gums;

• When the baby's bottom is red from diapers;

• When, for example, we are in tense and unpleasant situations such as going to the dentist, divorce proceedings, exams, driving tests, surgery, etc.;

The use of rescue remedies must not become a habit because they are for special mental conditions and not to solve a person's unreasonable lifestyle.

They are used depending on the situation. In emergency cases, drip 4 drops in a glass of water and drink in small sips until the state of shock passes, after which one sip is taken every 15, 30, or 60 minutes. If water or other drinks are not available at that time, they can be given undiluted, directly under the tongue. For unconscious persons, drops drip on the temples, behind the ear, in the mouth, or on the hand at the joint where the pulse is felt. Because of those places, the drops penetrate our bodies very quickly.

If it is necessary to give them for a long time, make a solution and give four drops four times a day.

They can also be used as a poultice, so six drops are soaked in half a litre of water. They can be applied to the external wound in the form of a cold or warm compress. Two pure, undiluted drops on the tongue are known to cure and restore consciousness in epilepsy and heart attacks within seconds. Granules can be used instead of liquids.

Other situations which we can use the rescue remedy are:

• In comatose states and when the patient is unconscious;

• Can be used for bites and stings;

• In cases of hair loss due to injury or psychological shock, use this remedy when you have bleeding or burns;

• For minor injuries, bites, muscle pain, redness of the skin, warts, bruises, psoriasis, bone pain, as an auxiliary medicine during massage, sprains, etc. Rescue cream can be used, which contains all the ingredients of the drops of the same name, plus crab apple, whose role is purification.

This cream can also be used by pregnant women if they are concerned about the appearance of their skin. The cream is also used for warts in the elderly and for barley on the eye.

Use of rescue remedies on animals: Rescue remedies can also be used on animals by adding 2-3 drops of Bach remedies to drinking water. If used, for example, for cows, add 10 drops to drinking water or more than 4 drops to 2 litres of water. For animals, if we don't know what to give, we should always give a rescue remedy.

If we have a dog that does not accept training or we need to move it, Walnut will help a lot. If we have one dog and get another, Walnut helps the dog adapt to the new situation. When we drive the dog in the car, so his vomiting is given a rescue remedy, plus Scleranthus. Even in this case, a therapeutic bottle with drops can be made and given more often.

If the animal constantly repeats the same mistakes, a chestnut bud is given. In cases of shock in animals, the Star of Bethlehem is given; in cases where the dog is untrustworthy, the Larch is given. If there is a fight with another animal or if there is a parasitic dog, a crab apple is given. For cleaning wounds in animals, a solution with crab apple is used, followed by rescue cream. If the dog is possessive, walks in front of our feet, behind our feet, and is always next to us, chicory is given. When animals are sick or recovering, Oliva is given to help them overcome the pain. Dogs can also be mischievous because they are afraid and can bite people because they have been hurt in the past. Then we give them Mimulus. The rule of consuming Bach flower remedies four times a day does not apply to animals because they drink water that is given to them more than once. Unless we know that they are not eating or drinking, we should make sure that they get four drops during the day.

Bach flower remedies are also used with plants and flowers. When we transplant flowers or change the country or place, we use walnut; when they freeze in the cold, we use rescue remedy; and so on. We put 3–4 drops in the water for watering. If they have green ears, we use crab apple and walnut. If we haven't watered them for a long time, they blame us, and they should be given Willow (5 drops in two litres of water for watering).

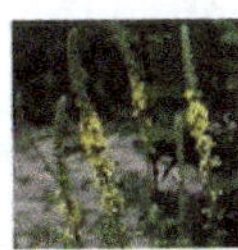

AGRIMONY – Agrimonia eupatorium

This Bach flower remedy is used for short-term conditions, such as mood swings. People who need this remedy behave carefree and satisfied in front of their surroundings, which is why it is a little more difficult to detect this condition. To every question asked, these people answer, "Thank you, I am great," which is not true at all because it is their mask in front of others around them. Very often, they say, "Only my soul knows how I feel."

These people are troubled by internal worries and fears such as financial problems, worries related to diseases, loss of money, problems at work, pain caused by other people, etc. They never talk about their problems in front of the people around them. They are always smiling, in a good mood, and very considerate of their surroundings, but there is no harmony within them. They hide their worries under the mask of laughter and humour. Instead of turning within themselves and solving their problems, these people run away in search of new ways of entertainment. They are always looking for company and do not want to be alone, because then they will have to face their problems and admit to themselves that the problem is in them. They like company because then they forget about what troubles them or about their worries, but they don't want to talk about it with the people around them. These are people who love peace; quarrels and unkindness disturb them, and they would do anything to avoid them. When they are sick, they do not pay attention to their condition.

People suffering from skin irritations and rheumatic diseases need agrimony. These are people who have hidden vices - drinking alcohol, smoking cigarettes - to forget about their problems and sufferings. They try to ignore the dark side of their lives and put on a mask of boldness and bravery (done persona).

• They get up at night and secretly eat from the fridge;

• They always leave a good impression on other people. They are constantly in motion, which is directed outside of themselves, in order to forget all the misery they have suppressed inside themselves. They like to work;

• They suffer from insomnia, are often tired, bite their nails, play with their hair, tremble, grind their teeth at night, and have irritated skin;

• Children feel lonely and sad. The medicine Agrimony will help them have better communication;

• It is used when a person has tendencies towards alcohol and cigarettes;

• These people have a strong sense of humour, which is why they are always at the centre of attention;

• They want to escape from the problems they have, so they resort to alcohol, drugs, parties, trips, etc.;

• They are used for severe pain, breathing disorders in asthma, and to improve appetite;

By using this remedy, people begin to see their problems, become objective, and begin to solve them. They become balanced, able to assess situations, and gain inner joy and cheerfulness.

Agrimony in combination with Scleranthus helps people who work night shifts - nursers, doctors, bakers, etc. - and also helps people who often change geographical zones, such as pilots, flight attendants, etc.

MitarM.'s healing experience with Bach Flower Remedy: Agrimony

When I faced internal conflicts and communication difficulties, Agrimony brought me relief. I began to feel open and able to express my true emotions and thoughts. This remedy helped me to get rid of the masks I was hiding behind and to find authenticity in my relationships.

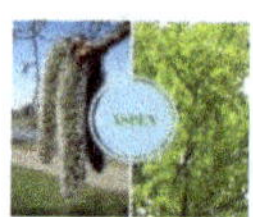

ASPEN – Populus tremula

This Bach flower remedy benefits people who have great fears that something terrible will happen. These people feel a fear that they cannot describe, and they do not know what they are afraid of. Fear for an unknown reason - fear that is unfounded - but with these people, the feeling of fear is great. People feel pulsations in the stomach area and tremors. They can't overcome that feeling of fear, and that's why even more fear arises. They have terrible premonitions; they are wet with sweat; they feel an internal tremor; and their skin crawls.

Aspen is prescribed for:

- Panic and unexplained fears of an impending disaster are often present;
- They feel panic and fear when they are alone, but this can also happen when they are in company;

- They are afraid to talk about their fears because they feel that people will laugh at them and think they are fools;
- They feel a mental fear that causes heart palpitations, tremors, and even loss of consciousness in a moment;

- Night terrors in children and adults;
- Sudden panic;
- They are afraid of evil spirits, ghosts, and have unreal imaginations, but at the same time they are enthusiastic about occult things;
- When this person happens to use narcotics, then they have horrible hallucinations;
- Aspen people are alcoholics who are obsessed with something;
- Aspen children usually want their room door open and the light on. They talk in their sleep, and they have nightmares. When they wake up, they are afraid to fall asleep again;
- When they have a panicky fear of the dark and strong premonitions;
- People who have a superstitious fear of magic should be given Aspen because they can become victims of their own magical illusions;

It is recommended to give Aspen the remedy for:

- Treatment of alcoholics as a supplement to therapy;

- In children who have been treated badly;
- In women who have been raped;
- Former drug addicts and people who participate in group meditations;

- Fear of invisible forces or inexplicable fear;

- Nightmarish dreams where you wake up in fear and panic;

- Fear of death and fear of thinking about religious topics;

- Fear of physical abuse;

- Fear of snakes and ghosts;

- Children who do not want to sleep alone in a dark room;

For people who are treated with Aspen, it is recommended to work in the garden, not consume alcohol, and avoid horror movies, as well as prolonged exposure to the sun's rays.

Affirmations that help with these conditions are:

• My heart is filled with hope and strength;

• I am in God's hands;

• I have a guardian angel.

Peter K.'s healing experience with Bach Flower Remedy: Aspen

Using Aspen was a transformative experience for me, giving me a profound sense of freedom from vague and inexplicable anxieties. Daily use has greatly reduced my sense of dread, allowing me to face life's uncertainties with a new calm. I have noticed a positive change in my overall emotional well-being, as Aspen has become a reliable companion in navigating the unknown aspects of life. In times of uncertainty, Aspen proved to be a gentle but powerful ally in promoting a sense of courage and inner strength within me.

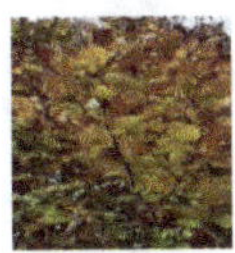

BEECH – Fagus sylvatica

Beech is most often a remedy for transient moods. A person who is a Beech type always finds fault with everyone and everything. She is always in a negative mood, and when she is in that mood, she is unable to see the positive side of the interlocutor. A person is nervous because of the behaviour of people around him, which is essentially a lack of tolerance, an inability to see the good side of the person across from us. The positive effect of this remedy is that it helps a person accept the people around him as they are. The threshold of tolerance and acceptance is at a high level. We have to be honest with ourselves. Well, we're not angels either, right?

They are most often prescribed to a person who:

• Does not approve of the weakness of the person across from him;

• Does not tolerate people who are frivolous;

• The habits and character of the person across from them can easily enrage them;

• These are people who want to order, dominate, and demand work, order, and discipline from everyone;

•They expect everyone to work and think like themselves;

• Lack of compassion;

• They do not accept the views of the people around them;

• They look for culprits and flaws; they are simply very limited;

• They do not recognise personal mistakes and shortcomings;

• They have a problem with food digestion;

• These are people who have been humiliated, so now they pay others back for it;

The beech remedy activates all that is positive in us, and at the same time, we are not burdened by small shortcomings. Because it has been scientifically proven that if we focus on negativity, it grows in us. This remedy helps a person see the beauty of life because they are not enjoying the moment because they are too busy judging the people around them. Beech removes stiffness in people.

Other situations where this remedy has a positive effect are:

• Intolerance and criticism. When a person judges others without walking part of the way in their shoes;

• When they see only negative things in their environment because they don't want to understand the reason why someone is unsuccessful in what they do;

• When a person has no tolerance for opinions that are not the same as theirs;

• When they lose their friends because of harsh language and communication;

These people want strictness, discipline, meticulousness, order, and punctuality without thinking and accepting that not everyone is the same and that we all have different attitudes towards the path we are going through, which is our life.

The description of the beech person is interesting: They look for shortcomings in others and do not look at their own shortcomings.

They hide behind a mask of arrogance and criticism. Due to their rigidity and internal tension, they often withdraw into themselves and isolate themselves from the environment.

A beech remedy helps a person to become measured, understandable, patient, tolerant, and to judge realistically.

Useful affirmations are:

• I am at peace with myself and others around me;

• I know that I know nothing.

Simon K.'s healing experience with Bach Flower Remedy: Beech

When I was prone to critical judgement and intolerance, the beech remedy taught me to accept other people with understanding and compassion. This remedy has helped me to develop a greater openness to differences and to approach others with love and support.

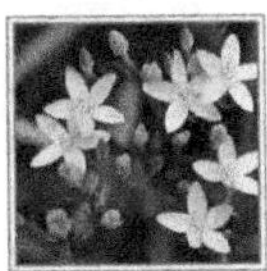

CENTAURY – Centaurium umbellatum

When a person needs this remedy, he is in such a good mood that he has the will to help everyone and do everything that someone would ask of him. This person does not know how to say no. The reason for this is that the person needs love and attention. They are afraid that if they say, "No, I don't have time for you," people won't like them anymore.

They are faithful listeners to other people's problems and often allow people around them to trample on them. But there comes a moment when the glass is over and the person flares up for no reason. Then the people around them are surprised, and often comment about them at that moment: "What happened to him? He was always so patient." They have a very hard time accepting this change.

Centaury teaches people to say no without remorse or discomfort. He will continue to help the people around him; he will listen to them, but he will know how to set a limit. They will learn to pay attention to themselves and say no without the other party getting angry and feeling offended. Their intuition becomes stronger, and they will know when to say no, according to the character of the interlocutor.

Centaury is prescribed for:

• People who suppress anger and store it in the jaw area;

• People who are weak-willed, good-natured, and pleasant, so others take advantage of them;

• People who are susceptible to other people's influences; follow the wishes of the people around them;

• People who give more than their means, thereby destroying their own lives;

• People who depend on family or work cannot break with the old and start a new path. Basically, they are very calm and kind people;

• When they lack the joy of life and their own life experience;

• Too attached to parents and family;

• Persons who cannot be proven as persons with their own attitude;

• People who voluntarily work to the point of exhaustion, like draft horses;

• During long-term and debilitating illnesses, when the patient's will gives way, Centaury gives new strength to the patient's spirit and body;

Centaury is needed by people who have problems with circulation or anaemia. These people can be influenced very easily; they have no vitality in them. They are hypersensitive and want to be recognized.

This type of child is good-natured, talkative, pleasant, and never causes problems for their parents. Praise and reprimands have a great impact on these children.

Adults are very easily influenced by people who are mentally stronger than them. An example of such a person is a middle-aged girl who is left alone without a family because she is caring for her old mother. Or a young mother who will do anything to please her son - a spoiled mama's boy.

These people often suffer from exhaustion and fatigue because they derive their strength from pleasing the people around them.

These are people who do not have their own opinion and always agree with other people's opinions; they allow everyone to shout at them because they are people with low self-esteem.

The centaury remedy is the most sensitive of all 38 Bach flower remedies. With this remedy, a person learns to make his own decisions and pay attention to his own life.

Jaroslav L.'s healing experience with Bach Flower Remedy: Centaury

As I often tended to take on other people's responsibilities and sacrifice my own needs, Centaury taught me to set boundaries and take care of myself. Through the use of this essence, I began to feel stronger and to express my needs without guilt. Centaury helped me develop greater self-esteem and confidence.

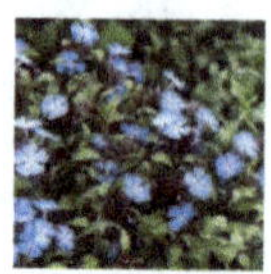

CERATO – Ceratostigma willmottianum

The vibration of this remedy relates to decision-making and inner security.

In this state, a person makes a decision, but immediately after making a decision, he begins to doubt its correctness, he begins to question other people about whether his decision is good, he receives a lot of information, and he becomes confused. In the end, he doesn't even know what his personal decision is.

This remedy is prescribed to people who:

• They cannot make their own decisions and act on them because other people's opinions have a great influence on them;

• Doubt themselves;

• People who go from one doctor to another and ask everyone for their opinion about their health and, in fact, have no use for it, collect information but do not use it;

• Children who are insecure and indecisive;

• People who are never satisfied with the advice they receive because it contradicts their opinion;

• People who are very talkative and constantly seek advice from others;

• People who have some clear ideas of their own, are intelligent, but do not have the courage to realise their ideas; that's why they go from one person to another, ask questions, and get contradictory answers, which confuses them;

• They live in a fantasy world;

• They uncritically accept all fad diets;

• It helps a person remember and clarify their dreams;

The Cerato remedy helps a person understand that he can make decisions on his own without consulting or influencing the opinions of other people. Intuition in these people often gives correct answers and insights, but in the real world, real thoughts and arguments do not give a person the strength to act in accordance with his intuition and his inner self. This creates conflict and inner uncertainty, which is very difficult for these people.

The most common question among these people is:

• What would you do if you were in my place?

They know the answer themselves, but they still can't rely on themselves, and the environment considers them limited personalities and maybe a little stupid.

Cerato remedies act on a person so that he becomes confident in himself, in his decisions, and in his thoughts. Then they become people who do not allow anyone or any arguments to sway them. After using the Cerato remedy, these people become wise, reasonable, and self-confident.

Useful affirmations in these situations are:

• Only I can decide what is good for me;

• I listen to my inner voice and trust it;

Christopher R.'s healing experience with Bach Flower Remedy: Cerato

When I was faced with indecision and a lack of faith in my own decisions, the Bach flower remedy Cerato provided me with inner security and determination. This remedy helped me discover and accept my inner wisdom and intuition, which always guided me to make the right decisions in life. Today I made decisions for myself, and I am proud of my choices.

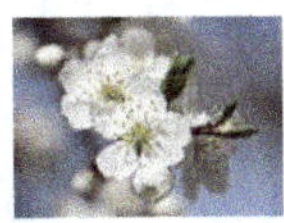

CHERRY PLUM – Prunus cerasifera

This is one of the Bach flower remedies contained in the rescue remedy for emergency care. It is a remedy for people who have great fears of losing control over their own actions, such as hysterical attacks. A person wants to do something that they would never normally do. These are situations that they later regret having done. In such a situation, they may have suicidal thoughts about themselves and the people around them. This is why this situation is really serious and requires treatment. The person cannot help himself; he is in deep despair. He has the feeling that he is on the verge of a nervous breakdown and that he will go crazy.

This Bach flower remedy is prescribed for people:

• Have a fear of losing internal control, an urge for violence, or a nervous breakdown;

• Great fear that their mind is overloaded;

• Hopelessness and deep depression in those people who suffer from mental and physical agony for a long time. They have the feeling that their brains will explode from the tension and effort;

• In people who, in a fit of rage, beat their children and throw objects at them;

• During hysterical shouting and cursing;

• When people lack emotional control due to obsession with fears and despair;

• These personalities are constantly stretching and showing restlessness within themselves;

• They always hide their fears from others around them;

• Persons who were tortured;

• People who have crazy ideas and psychoses, as well as those who have already been treated for these conditions and feel a great fear that they will return to the hospital again;

• Tendency to commit suicide;

• Drug addiction;

•Parkinson's and other neurological diseases;

• People who were in the war;

With great success, this remedy helps children who urinate at night (they control themselves so much during the day that when they sleep, they express their fears by wetting the bed). It is also given to children who have tantrums - they throw themselves on the floor, hit their heads against the wall, etc. A fantastic essence that helps children who, for example, become hysterical because they don't get everything they want (rescue remedies can also be given). This is also a thyroid-balancing remedy.

Very often, these people know how to say:

• I feel like I'm sitting on a powder keg, and I'm going to explode at any moment.

• I am terrified of my thoughts; the thought comes to me to take a knife and kill my wife (husband).

These people have too much fear of going crazy and losing self-control; their nerves are terribly tense, and they are afraid of doing something terribly bad that they will regret for the rest of their lives.

The cherry plum remedy works by increasing mental endurance, calming a person, encouraging them, and leading to mental stability. An example is giving this remedy to a woman who is recovering from a serious illness, has hysterical attacks, and lacks mental control. This remedy gives her calmness, strength, and courage to open up to life and bring calmness and spontaneity into her life.

Mona J.'s healing experience with Bach Flower Remedy: Cherry Plum

When I was faced with intense emotional stress and felt out of control, the Cherry Plum remedy became my saviour. This remedy helped me get rid of internal pressure and anxiety. I started to feel calmer and able to think rationally even in the most difficult situations. Using the cherry plum remedy made me feel strong and confident in taking control of my emotions and making wise decisions.

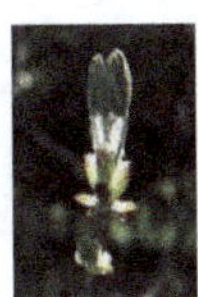

CHESTNUT BUD – Aesculus sp.

People who need Bach flower remedies for chestnut bud are those who keep making the same mistakes without realising it. And not understanding this problem themselves, they are powerless to make any change. It is the remedy that wakes us up from "sleep" and allows us to see the mistake in ourselves and not repeat that action or behaviour. It helps us to understand that we should observe and learn from other people's mistakes, because only then will life not slap us and we will live easily and contentedly.

This Bach flower remedy is prescribed for:

• Absence, lack of concentration, and inability to learn from their own mistakes (because they quickly forget what happened);

• People who are two steps ahead with their minds than their actions;

• A person running away from the past;

• Physically ill persons with occasional relapses (example: migraine attacks that repeat during a conversation with the same person);

• People who lack self-awareness;

• Lack of concentration;

• People who accept new things very quickly;

• Weak and slow learning; forgetfulness;

• Children who are impatient, careless, and undisciplined lack progress and development;

With chestnut bud remedies, we treat children who are often distracted and inattentive and do not notice some things around them. An example of this is a child who often forgets a sandwich for school, writes incorrectly during dictation, and lags behind other students.

Parents often say about their child: "My child is a little behind; he is late compared to his friends." And at the same time, they do not notice that at that moment, their child lives in his own world (another time and space). If they forcibly return the child to normal reality, they achieve the opposite effect: the child becomes more and more insecure about himself and his actions.

The chestnut bud remedy fantastically helps align inner thoughts with material action.

Mary F.'s healing experience with Bach Flower Remedy:

Chestnut Bud

When I was prone to repeating the same mistakes and stagnating in my development, the Chestnut Bud remedy gave me the awareness to learn from the past and see my mistakes that I was repeating. This remedy has helped me develop a greater awareness of my behaviour patterns and open myself up to new experiences and learning.

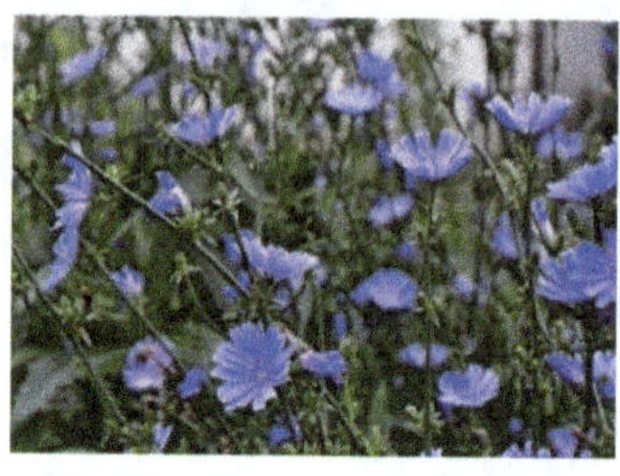

CHICORY – Cichorium sp.

This Bach flower remedy is the vibration for transitory moods. In this mood, the person looks like he wants to own someone; he is possessive. He loves people, but it's selfish love. Most often, these people say to you, "I love you, if..."Their love is related to conditioning. An example of this can be parents who, when a child separates from them and has his own life, say, "Don't leave; it's not fair to you." Another example is when a mother expects her children to come to lunch every week, and if it doesn't happen, she gets angry and offended and tries to manifest it emotionally. She simulates an illness to manipulate them and get their attention. These are very simple and everyday examples of Chicory people behaving possessively, looking for love, but in the wrong ways. And they will never get it because the environment starts to treat them with anger and maybe abandon them.

Chicory flower remedy is prescribed for:

• People full of egoism, self-pity, and desire for supremacy;

• Selfish people who want the world to revolve around them and do everything to draw attention to themselves. They often say, "Nobody loves me";

• People who love others and selflessly protect them without asking for any favours for themselves;

• Taking too much care of a sick person (e.g., a woman who takes care of her husband who is suffering from cancer and is too worried);

• Uneducated, crying children who do not want to be alone. These are children who cry and do stupid things just to get attention; sometimes they get sick;

• Possessive children who don't go anywhere without their mom (Holly helps in this case);

• Possessive motherly love;

• With judges who should be objective;

• With deep inner dissatisfaction due to a lack of love The person feels a deep inner emptiness and dissatisfaction and has the feeling that he has never been loved;

When escaping from illness in ancient Egypt, chicory was considered a medicine for the liver. Chicory type people want everyone to submit to them, and if they don't get it, they start to feel sorry for themselves. They have a fear of losing friends, a feeling that no one loves them, that they have been deceived. Most often, they run into illness to attract attention. When their expectations are not met, these people get angry and assume the role of a martyr.

This remedy is also used for:

• People who cry because of the instability of the environment;

• People who, while doing a service, immediately ask for a return service;

• People who want to keep the ones they love to themselves so they can control their lives. They criticise their lifestyle or the way they do things;

• Individuals who become very angry if they do not receive the attention they feel is their right;

• With the neurotic behaviour of people who, in order to get what they want, use all possible means and tricks: self-pity, tears, and finally anger. An example is a person who faints in order to attract and retain attention;

• A child may pretend to have a stomach-ache just to get attention;

• A mother who gives in to her child and lies to herself that it is love, but it is only a way to stay close to him;

• A person who constantly demands attention;

• Selfishness;

• People who consume large amounts of wine;

• Manipulative, critical, self-centred people who want attention;

• Hysteria;

• Too many expectations from other people;

• Self-promotion to attract attention;

• Internal void;

• Childhood without love and attention;

• Attention-seeking mother (the attention-seeking child is Heather);

An example of chicory children are those sweet children who get everything they want, but the first time they don't get something, they start screaming to get attention and get what they want.

With this remedy, people learn how to accept others and give them freedom. They learn how to give without expecting anything in return. After using this essence, a person becomes warm and in a good mood, with a feeling of security and protection that also transfers to the environment.

Jane J.'s healing experience with Bach Flower Remedy:

Chicory

When I was overwhelmed with concern for others and prone to manipulative behaviour, Bach flower remedy Chicory taught me true love, which is tender, unconditional, and unbiased. This remedy helped me develop healthier relationships with others, with greater freedom and respect for the environment.

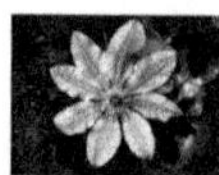

CLEMATIS – Clematis sp.

This Bach flower remedy is for people who are absent in spirit, looking at something or someone but not noticing it. It is often found in children at school when the teacher is teaching, but they seem not to be there with their minds. But not only in children; it can appear very often in adults as well. It seems that they are dreaming with their eyes open; they are not in the present but in a fantasy, an illusion about the future. For example, while driving a car, we think about something else and suddenly realise that we have reached our destination, but we are not aware of the course of the drive.

The Clematis remedy is prescribed for:

• People who participate less in real life and are closed to their fantasy world;

• People who have little energy on a physical level;

• They complain of cold feet and hands; and they are pale; their heads are empty. For example, he goes to the kitchen and forgets why he came there. Or adults who often say, I can't feel the circulation in my legs, I can't feel my body from the middle down, etc;

• People who are dreamers want to escape from reality;

• People who can fall asleep in any position, for example, sitting on a chair. They have a great need for sleep, but it is not because they are tired; here, the soul wants to escape to some world of imagination where they would feel at home;

• They cannot accept reality; they fall asleep with the TV on, and while they are at mass in the church, they also fall asleep;

• In cases of indifference, deconcentration, or lethargy;

• For people who are sick and don't want to move a little finger to get better (example: given to a 12-year-old girl who had too many freckles on her face, and because of that, she was very unhappy, lost self-confidence, and became withdrawn and very quiet);

• In people who use neuroleptics and narcotics;

• People who dream during the day and their thoughts are somewhere far away, do not pay attention to what is happening around them, are distracted and isolated;

• People who react equally to bad and good news or events;

• People who do not strive for a quick recovery during illness because they have a weak instinct for self-help;

• People who wait until they die in order to meet those they love who are already deceased;

• When people want to be alone with their thoughts;

• In complete loss of interest in life and work;

• Lack of ambition;

• In cases of fainting, coma;

• Lack of desire to live, suicidal thoughts;

• In cases of sterility;

Clematis helps a person to ground himself in the present, in the moment in which he lives, in a certain moment, to be truly where he is with his mind. These people rarely show fear or aggression. Many people who are involved in spirituality need Clematis to balance their physical and mental selves. It also helps with better concentration on the exam because the person is down-to-earth and realistic.

Dr. Bach calls the state of Clematis "a decent and fine form of suicide." These people have great creative gifts, which is why we often meet them in the world of fashion, film, writing, etc.

This remedy successfully helps people who live in the hope of a better future, hoping that "their 5 minutes" will come. And in fact, with such thinking, they miss the beauty of the present moment of living. Very often, these people say, "When I have to face something unpleasant or ugly, I retreat into my own world."

The clematis remedy helps to improve concentration, restore interest and strength in life, and lead to new victories.

An affirmation that helps in these situations:

• I understand more and more the dependence between inner peace and the outer world.

Marko P.'s healing experience with Bach Flower Remedy:

Clematis

When I was prone to daydreaming, fantasising, and being absent from the present moment and surroundings, Clematis helped me connect with my inner creativity and focus. This Bah flower remedy brought me a sense of greater presence in the present and concentration, which made me more productive and inspired.

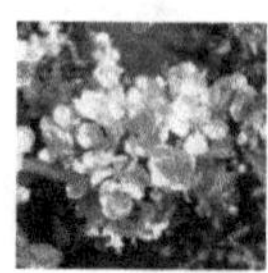

CRAB APPLE – Malus sylvestris

The remedy of crab apple can be a personality type or a cure for a fleeting mood. It is associated with order, purity, and perfection. It is a remedy for physical and mental purification. It has a purifying effect on the physical and mental levels and is therefore often used in combination with other remedies, especially for the treatment of skin diseases. These are people who pay too much attention to details and little things. They pay too much attention to details; they don't see the whole situation. An example is people who constantly clean the house; they are too meticulous and want everything to be perfect. For them, the home must always be the way they arrange it. For example, they wait impatiently for their guests to leave so they can arrange the pillows on the bed after them.

Often, these people have a feeling of impurity in themselves, on a physical or emotional level. They have sinful and dirty thoughts. They start hating themselves. When they look in the mirror, they often say, "Oh my God, I'm so ugly," they put themselves on a lower level than others, they think they are not smart enough, etc. They lack a sense of self-acceptance, just the way they are.

Bach flower remedy Crab apple is prescribed for:

• People who hate themselves;

• People who have lost their sense of many things in life;

• To cleanse the soul of bad thoughts and habits;

• As an assistant in weight loss diets;

• To eliminate cold symptoms, remove secretions from the upper respiratory tract;

• Purification of the organism from excessive intake of antibiotics;

• During pregnancy, when a woman vomits a lot (a walnut and rescue remedy can be added here);

• For flowers when transplanting;

• In cases of fear of wrongly prescribed medicines;

• Cleaning the skin of warts, eczema, infections, and gallstones;

• When children stutter, they cannot speak fluently;

• For purulent acne, (mix 4 drops of crab apple with olive oil and rub around the acne and on it);

• For people who think they have an illness. For example, if they see a pimple, they immediately think they have skin cancer;

• To clear the barley in the eye;

• During painful periods;

• People who are overweight and do not accept themselves go on strict diets and lose more and more pounds. They constantly find flaws in their appearance. They don't like themselves (e.g., they have too much acne, or they don't like their hair, etc.);

• With perfectionists;

• Fear of infections;

These people wash their hands too often. Even though everything is clean at home, they clean everything all the time. They are afraid that if they don't clean the windows, they will get some disease or infection. This essence has great success in the treatment of anorexia when the person's only thought is, I am too fat. In this case, other remedies are added, and it is very important to know how the person experienced this state, the state of the family, the marriage of their parents, the attitude of their parents towards them, etc. For example, crab apples can be given, but if they are too principled and do not eat the food they need, they fall out of balance.

Crab Apple helps to remove negative views from life.

It helps people get back into balance, live their lives in harmony, and start loving themselves exactly as they are. People become generous. Meditation helps with this personality type.

Risto H.'s healing experience with Bach Flower Remedy:

Crab Apple

I was at a point in my life where I felt dirty, uncomfortable, and unhappy with my physical appearance. Crab apple brought me a sense of physical and emotional purity. This remedy healed me from the inside and helped me accept my own authenticity - that I am worth just the way I am.

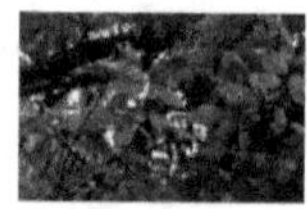

ELM – Ulmus sp.

People who have the characteristics of the Elm remedy have a sense of great responsibility within themselves. They usually do very responsible jobs and are successful in their work. The negative side of these types of people is that they take on too much responsibility; they think they can do everything at once. The moment they realise that they are overloaded with obligations, they feel too much pressure because of it and cannot cope with the situation. In general, these are capable people who are hardworking, intuitive, and selflessly work for the community.

This remedy is prescribed for:

• Feelings of immaturity for too much responsibility and obligation;

• The feeling that someone has been betrayed (an example is a doctor who feels that he has betrayed his patients);

• Fatigue due to too many obligations; they do not have the strength to complete upcoming tasks;

• People who suddenly fall into depression, despair, and fear whether they will be able to find a way out of the situation they are in;

Elm remedies are characterised as "weak moments in the lives of strong people."

These are people inclined to altruism, maximally devoted to work, not realising that their strength is limited. This condition is often encountered during menopause. People forget that everyone is responsible for themselves and that they must first fulfil the needs of their soul and then the expectations of the people around them.

Bach flower remedy elm helps a person to become calmer, more settled, and to ask himself why he took on all these responsibilities. Also, the remedy helps a person gain the strength to complete all tasks. These are people who have found their place in life, know their abilities, and know where they are going. They follow their purpose and choices in life and want to do something good for humanity. With the vibration of this Bach flower remedy, people become confident and trustworthy. They understand that they should include several stages of rest in planning their duties.

Jelena K.'s healing experience with Bach Flower Remedy:

Elm

At a time in my life when I was faced with too many responsibilities and obligations and felt overwhelmed, Elm gave me the strength to face those challenges. This remedy helped me find a balance between obligations and personal needs, which created a greater sense of self-confidence and success in work and private life.

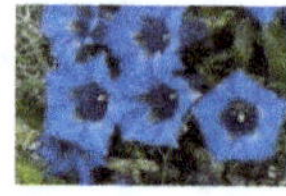

GENTIAN – Gentiana sp.

The vibration of the Gentian remedy is associated with states of disappointment and discouragement, doubt, dejection, and weakness that occur as a result of defeat or disappointment. These people lose faith very quickly if something unpleasant happens to them, and they are immediately disappointed. An unpleasant event can be a failure in life or a failure in an exam. They believe that all difficulties in life are the result of their fate and not their negative attitudes. Even if they have short-term success, they come back and give up. For them, this is not a state of deep depression but a surface depression when they succumb momentarily.

This Bach flower remedy is prescribed for:

• States of sadness whose reasons are not clear;

• Depression of unknown cause;

• Pessimistic people who see only the negative side of things;

• People for whom every obstacle is insurmountable, even though it is easy to overcome it;

• People who lack faith;

•When people are very worried and expect the worst to happen, for example, they will lose their job;

• They doubt everything, they don't believe;

• He does not believe in the universe, in God;

• Hypochondria;

• During menopause;

• When a person loses his job and finances;

• In cases of despondency and depression for known reasons, such as the death of a close family member;

• Children of divorced parents, children with bad grades in school, and elderly people in homes for the elderly;

• Loss of official position;

• Passivity;

• Despondency in the process of recovery from illness. If there is a relapse, they think it is the end of the world, and they are discouraged;

The vibration of this flower remedy has great success with children who become timid and do poorly in school, with young people who break up with girls and become mentally ill, or with children who quarrel with friends.

People who belong to the Gentian remedy type have an internal blockage at the soul level, due to which they do not believe in the action of Dr. Bach's remedies. A person wants to believe but cannot; he thinks, analyses, and decides, but always suppresses the result inside himself. Gentian helps them live with the conflicts they have within. It gives them strength and courage to try again where they failed.

Gentian, in combination with crab apple, works very successfully for children who wet the bed at night. Adults in Gentian states are helped by reading books such as The Power of the Subconscious or How Thoughts Work.

Maria F.'s healing experience with Bach Flower Remedy:

Gentian

My experience with the Bach flower remedy Gentian has been very positive. When I faced depression and pessimism, Gentian reminded me that the universe is full of possibilities and that I should not lose hope. I felt braver and more open to new possibilities; I succeeded where I was sure I would not succeed.

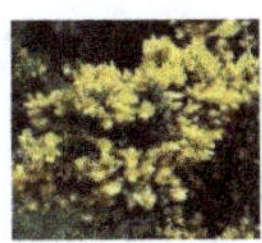

GORSE – Ulex europaeus

Bach flower remedy Gorse is used as a remedy for transient moods. It is actually the next state after Gentian, which is called hopelessness. In this state, a person does not see hope in life and does not see a bright spot at the end of the tunnel. These people often say to themselves,"There is no hope for me" or "I give up; I don't fight anymore." They need a lot of motivation from their family. However, there is a situation when they will refuse any help and say"Why are you harassing me?"I came to the doctor because you made me, not because I wanted to." In these situations, hopelessness, doubt, and despair arise, and these people think that no one and nothing can help them.

The Gorse remedy is prescribed for:

• People who consider their unhappiness to be fate, hereditary, or congenital;

• Chronic patients to start treatment that would give them hope;

• Lack of ambition;

• Melancholy;

• People who allow other people to persuade them against their will; With people who constantly say, What will it do to me? I've tried everything, but it's no use;

• Helps with the last stage of a disease, for example, cancer;

• In people who move away from their own selves;

• people who expect healing from the outside but cannot understand that healing is happening inside us;

• Chronic diseases in the early stages;

• Depression and inner fatigue. Often people say to you,"I asked everything, but..." or"It doesn't make sense...".

These people are hopeless and often suffer from some chronic disease. Or they have been treated unsuccessfully many times, and doctors have explained to them that they will never fully recover. They try therapy again, but inside they are convinced that it does not help. They often have a yellow or pale waxy face colour and dark rings around the eyes. The positive effect of the vibration of this flower remedy is that it gives hope and emotionally lifts the person out of the darkness, whereby the person accepts the therapy and is motivated to seek help. It allows him to be convinced to start the treatment again and not be disappointed at the first failure. People treated with the Gorseremedy begin to believe in the positive results of the treatment. They finally realise that hopelessness is a brake on the healing process.

Useful affirmations for these conditions:

•"Hope is medicine";

• "Every new day is a new opportunity."

Marinela H.'s healing experience with Bach Flower Remedy:

Gorse

Gorse gave me a lot of support when I felt lost and listless. The greatest support and help came at a time when I thought there was no hope for me. His energy gave me hope and faith that there is always light at the end of the tunnel. I felt encouraged and ready to face challenges.

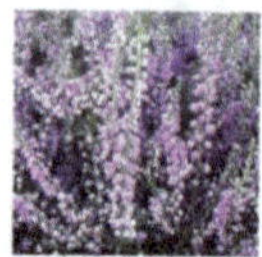

HEATHER – Calluna vulgaris

Bach flower remedy Heather is depicted in people who are focused only on themselves, selfish people who always complain about their lives, saying that they are very unhappy or sick. These people know how to make an elephant out of a fly, as our grandmothers would say. When they are in that state, they are not interested in the suffering of the people around them. They do not pay the slightest attention to the problems of the interlocutor. They have the need to constantly tell their story and to complain, which is why the people around them avoid them, and the reason is that they cannot listen to the same story over and over again.

These people get very close to you, whisper to you, try to touch you, or hold your hand or sleeve while talking to you. If you look away for a moment, the person will call you by name, so you look at them and pay attention to their words. They want to get rid of their thoughts by sharing them with you and always focusing the conversation on themselves.

The Heather remedy is prescribed for:

• People who talk all the time, talk fast, and no one can take their turn;

• They want to be the centre of attention;

• They don't want to be alone because they live off the vitality and energy of the people around them;

• Possessive persons who subtly and imperceptibly dominate and are possessive;

• They pretend to be martyrs, but they only care about themselves;

• They are obsessed with problems and diseases;

• Single mother;

• An adult in the emotional state of a child often says, "I was a poor child", just like small children who need attention and kindness from their surroundings;

• Too worried about themselves, their problems, and their illnesses;

Every person can fall into such a state at some point in their life. Often, these are people who come from cold families where they have been deprived of emotional warmth since birth. These are people who live off the energy of others around them, which is why it's scary for them when they're alone.

In order to get rid of such people, we have to act brutally because they don't leave their victims alone so easily. It doesn't matter who they talk to; it can be an unknown person.

Heather people are "energy vampires" who come up to you, talk to you, and actually drain your vital energy, so that after talking to them, you feel completely drained.

By using the remedy, Heather, people realise that others have problems that they want to share with someone. They learn not only to speak but also to listen, and thus they will actually get the attention they are missing so much. They begin to participate in solving the problems of the world around them. They gain self-confidence and courage.

Robert W.'s healing experience with Bach Flower Remedy:

Heather

Heather taught me the value of learning to listen and care for others. The vibration of this Bach flower remedy taught me to be considerate and compassionate towards others. Today I feel happier and more fulfilled because I, too, can help others.

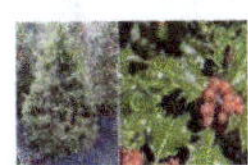

HOLLY – Ilex aquifolium

Bach flower remedy Holly has the most negative vibration of all 38 flower remedies. It is associated with hatred, jealousy, suspicion, envy, mistrust, and great anger. Holly is described as a mood state because we all feel angry or jealous at times. In that state, we can only hurt someone, and we cannot give love. The vibration of this remedy helps a person accept love and be able to return it. Dr. Bach says about the vibration of this flower remedy: Holly opens human hearts to love and kindness.

Holly is most often prescribed for:

• Negative people, pessimists who see small obstacles in life as big problems;

• In cases of stagnation or stopping during treatment, Holly helps prolong the healing process. Holly is given to impulsive people and calm people;

• people who are callous, disaffected, and have a desire for revenge;

• Resentment;

• An unhappy person for no reason;

• Cruelty to other people, aggression, malice, envy;

• A holly person who is energetic and active;

• It has a beneficial effect on terminally ill, incurable diseases;

• people who feel isolated, rejected, and abandoned;

• With intellectuals who are fighting for prestige;

• In case Dr. Bach's flower remedies have no effect, Holly is given;

• For children, when a second child is born in the family;

• With envy on all levels, with fear of fraud, and with people who constantly complain about other people;

A person of the Holly type is not understanding, is angry, has a bad character, is irritable, and all this leads to unhappiness and feelings of insecurity. They fight alone for the existence of their feelings.

When a child is born, it learns to give and receive love. If this is taken away from him, he falls into severe disappointment and begins to defend himself and isolate himself. Love is a great force, but its opposite is very negative. When these negative feelings prevail, such as hatred, jealousy, malice, and the like, they become a serious cause of central ailments.

After using the vibration of the Holly remedy, a person begins to live in inner harmony and love, deeply understands the feelings of others, and rejoices in the successes of others around him.

65

Zara M.'s healing experience with Bach Flower Remedy:

Holly

Holly helped me deal with negative emotions like jealousy and anger. His energy brought me inner peace and helped me find kindness in myself and compassion for others. Now I feel balanced and harmonious. I'm happy.

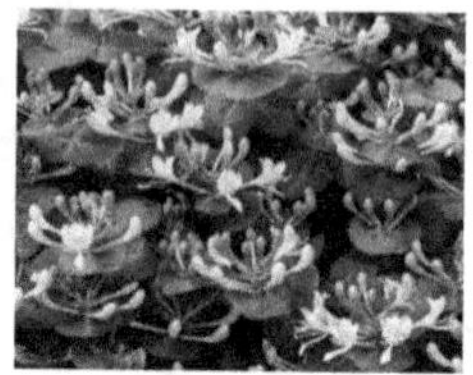

HONEYSUCKLE – Lonicera caprifolium

This remedy can be a personality type or a cure for a fleeting mood. Problems with these people arise due to weak internal motivation and a lack of initiative. A person in this state is mentally in another time and place, which makes him incapable of action. In this state, the person does not allow himself to be guided by himself according to the needs of his soul. The vibration of this remedy is related to the feeling when a person longs for the past, or rather lives in the past.

The vibration of this remedyis prescribed for:

• When a person returns to images, memories, or accidents from the past;

• After experiencing shock, after which the images come back without stopping;

• in people who idealise the past;

• In workers, migrants, or migrants travelling home; sadness or nostalgia for the homeland;

• Grief due to the death of a close person (they cannot accept it, and they constantly live in the memories);

• Regret unfulfilled dreams;

• Weak interest in current problems, because their thoughts are in the past;

• They often say, "It seems like yesterday...";

• For a woman who cannot establish a new relationship after the death of her husband;

• For older actresses who are stuck in a time when they were very popular;

• With older people who constantly talk about how it used to be much nicer;

• Situations in which people regret missed opportunities, unfulfilled wishes, lost hope, the painful realisation that something was not done right, but without feeling guilty about it;

• People who live in past accidents or situations and suffer as a result mentally and physically;

• People who lose all interest in the present;

• People who live from memories and don't expect anything more than what they already have;

• They suppress the fear of aging;

• People who ignore change;

• They reject the inner guidance, themselves;

• In people on their deathbed;

Dr. Bach said that the remedy of the honeysuckle flower can expel from a person's head all the anger, sadness, and worries from the past. These people do not want to accept the new developments. They escape into the past in order not to face problems in the present.

This remedy helps people to learn from the past, to be in active contact with it, but not to cling senselessly to the past.

Irene F.'s healing experience with Bach Flower Remedy:

Honeysuckle

Honeysuckle taught me to live in the present moment and accept life's changes. It freed me from being tied to the past and helped me open up to new possibilities. I feel liberated and can boldly move forward in life.

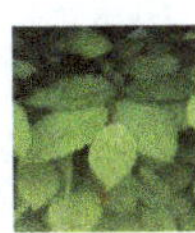

HORNBEAM – Carpinus betulus

This remedy can be a personality type or a mood type. A person feels tired and exhausted, but this is only the state of the person's mind. This condition can be temporary (transient) or chronic.

A transient condition can occur in students who study a lot before exams or when a person has a fracture and has to lie in bed for a long time, and when he has to move, he thinks he is not mentally ready for it.

A chronic condition is when a person, who constantly watches television and is less physically active, receives more information than he can mentally process.

These are the people who have a hard time waking up in the morning to start the day, but when they get up later, everything goes easily for them. Often in the morning, they say, "Just 5 more minutes to sleep." They are always late for work. While they sleep for another 5 minutes in the morning, they are mentally active and have a whole plan for that day. That's why they get exhausted, and when they wake up, they feel as tired as if they were digging a field. This is the reason why waking up in the morning is very difficult for them.

This remedy is prescribed for:

• People who feel physically and mentally exhausted are people who cannot bear the burden of everyday life;

• In cases of excessive psychological fear associated with daily activities;

• When they are tired in the morning and constantly complain of chronic fatigue, for example, people who say, "Who will go to work on Monday?"

• During the rehabilitation of drug addicts;

• With a feeling of heaviness in the head;

• Buzzing in the head after watching TV for a long time;

• In people who wake up more tired in the morning than in the evening when they go to sleep;

• Those people who think that they do not have enough mental and physical strength to carry the burden of life that is placed before them;

• It seems to them that they have too many daily obligations, but in fact, they manage to fulfil their obligations. It is more of a mental than a physical weakness;

• Liver diseases;

• Without strength, they are insecure and indecisive;

• As a poultice in patients with varicose veins;

• Rehabilitation;

•Hornbeam cladding is recommended for tired and irritated eyes;

These people spend their lives on precisely defined paths, and their free time is filled with inner restlessness and tension. Hornbeam gives them vitality and inner strength. These are often people who drink a lot of coffee, tea, and other stimulants. It is interesting that the Hornbeam type's fatigue disappears if something different happens, so they move from routine to other spheres.

Hornbeam is also used for plants; it gives vitality and energy to weak plants.

Hornbeam restores strength to those who have difficulty getting up in the morning and makes it easier for them to start the day.

A helpful thought in this state: "Joy is wisdom, and wisdom is joy."

Magdalena I.'shealing experience with Bach Flower Remedy:

Hornbeam

Hornbeam supported me when I faced fatigue or a lack of motivation. When I had a hard time waking up in the morning and starting the day and my duties, his energy refreshed me and gave me new strength to continue. Every morning, I feel full of energy and ready for new challenges. I start the day with ease and carry out my daily duties.

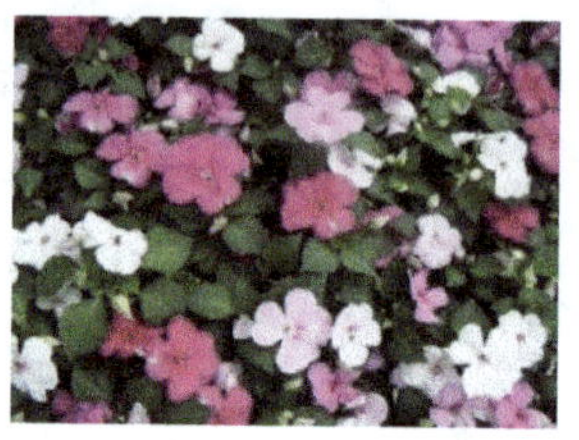

IMPATIENS – Impatiens sp.

This remedy is for the type of person who, due to excessive inner tension, is very irritable towards the environment. Everything they do, they do quickly, e.g., talk fast, walk fast, etc. They are impatient and do not understand people who are slower than them. They finish other people's sentences, have no patience, can't wait, and take work out of the hands of slower people around them. The slowness of the people around them annoys them. The impatient type of person is impatient, cannot be controlled, wastes energy everywhere, and ends up in a stressful situation.

The vibration of this remedy is prescribed for:

• People who are careless and prone to accidents;

• People with internal tension, emotional tension, impatience, and irritability;

• For people who constantly want to argue, want to criticise others, and constantly want to blame them for some situations;

• To people who know everything better than others and don't have the patience and nerves to explain. They often say, "While I explain to them, I will do the work myself."

• In people who react quickly to criticism and immediately get annoyed, even if the criticism is spoken diplomatically, they quickly calm down;

• People who solve everything quickly;

• Children who cry, rage, and want to take everything when they go shopping;

• Parents who quickly lose patience in raising children;

• People who constantly shake their legs or tap their fingers;

• Children who cannot fall asleep peacefully;

• Internal tension that can lead to spastic pains in different parts of the body. For example, colic after anger or rash after anger;

• In patients who state that they are tired, irritable, and angry with everything and everyone they come into contact with;

• For pain;

• Intolerance;

• Sudden cramping pain due to tension;

• Independent persons;

• Extroverted personalities;

• Impetuous, reckless people;

• Children who fight all the time;

• People who want to work alone;

People who need the Impatiens remedy vibration learn and understand new ideas very quickly and often know the end of a sentence before the other person finishes it. When they are sick and their healing does not progress quickly, they become nervous and irritable. Inner turmoil makes them unrestrained and careless. If they do not get rid of their inner nervousness by moving or walking, rashes, itching, reddening of the skin, etc. may appear.

The vibration of Impatiens will not slow these people down, but it will help them to concentrate on one thing and not to do several things at once. By vibrating the Impatiens essence, they will be able to optimally use their potential.

Vladimir M's healing experience with Bach Flower Remedy:

Impatiens

Impatiens remedy brought me calmness and patience at times when I was impatient or stressed. His energy slowed me down and taught me to appreciate the moment. Now I feel calm and balanced. I accept people who are slower than me, as long as we work together.

impatient or stressed. His energy slowed me down and taught me to appreciate the moment. Now I feel calm and balanced. I accept people who are slower than me, as long as we work together.

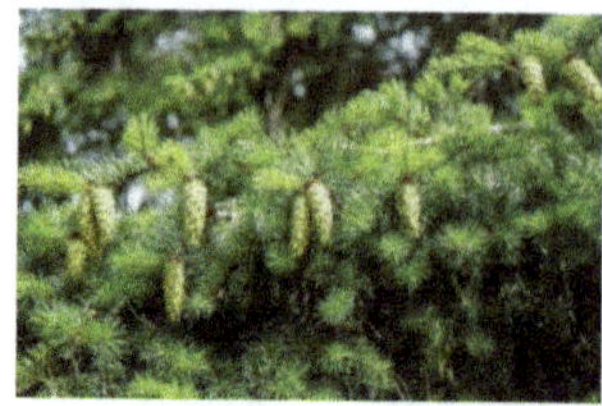

LARCH – Larix decidua

The vibration of the Bach flower remedy larch is associated with a lack of self-confidence. In that state, the healer, before starting to do something, says, "I know I won't succeed in this; it won't work out, so...". They are pre-concentrated on failure, and it is normal that they will experience failure. They have no faith in themselves, easily lose courage, and give up in every situation. They have an inferiority complex that has been hidden since childhood, although in fact they are often more capable than other people.

This vibration of the Bach flower remedy,larch,is prescribed for:

• Children who lack self-confidence in school or sports and therefore want to run away from school;

• Self-conscious people who often calmly accept the knowledge that they are losers;

• People who often say they can't...

• Distrust before the exam, divorce, anticipation of failure;

• Children who are afraid and want their parents to do everything for them;

• With alcoholism, when a person drinks to forget that he is not as capable as others;

• When people feel worthless and useless;

• Complexes of low value;

These people see the successes of others and wonder why they fail. They like being below the level of others and don't decide on things they think they can't handle (e.g., the possibility of professional development). They do not envy other people's success; they are interested in what others do; they praise them, but they feel and admit that they could not do it. They do not allow their inner selves to stand out. They cannot understand that success and failure are equally valuable in life.

This remedy makes a person decisive. Larch gives them the opportunity to try something new and see if it will work or not. The vibration of the Larch remedy helps a person focus on success.

Marian E.'s healing experience with Bach Flower Remedy:

Larch

Larch taught me to believe in myself and my abilities. When I was dealing with low self-esteem, Larch helped me and reminded me that I am capable of achieving anything I put my mind to. I feel confident and brave. I believe and am determined that I will succeed.

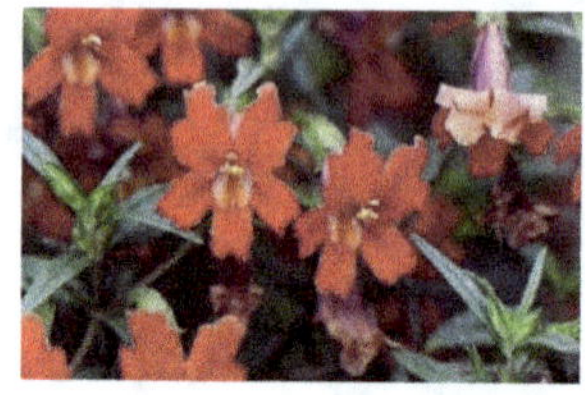

MIMULUS – Mimulus sp.

The Bach flower remedy mimulus has a red but also a yellow colour and illuminates the hopelessness that a person feels. It is the remedyfor fears of known origin. For example, when people are afraid of going to the dentist or are afraid of spiders, etc. If we know how to name our fear, then the remedy is Mimulus. This remedy is associated with the fear of the dark. Dr. Bach believes that these are the remains of the newborn's original fear of the outside world.

If it is a type of person, then they are shy, blush easily, get stressed at unexpected sounds, do not want to be in the company of people (e.g., at a party), and say,"I have work to do, I can't". They don't come. They don't want to be the centre of attention. They are blocked and afraid of saying something stupid; they don't know how to behave or what to say. Bach flower remedy Mimulusis prescribed for:

• Fear of public speaking is, for them, stress;

• Fear of familiar things; nervousness with everyday fears; difficult circumstances in everyday life;

• Stage fright;

• Abdominal cramps;

• Fear of the onset of illness, death;

• Fear of being alone; fear of being alive;

• In cases of illness, if the pains become stronger or if they do not go away;

• Crying in small children;

• Nightmares;

• Fear of unknown people;

• Phobia of the dark;

• Loss of friends, illness, pain, abuse, etc.;

• In children with a fear of the dark;

• When a child is shy and does not want to socialise with other children, he is afraid;

• Fear of being alone and fear of all kinds of sounds;

For example, if a child who suffers from asthma is nervous and afraid of unknown people, mimulus and agrimony are successful in solving breathing problems.

People who need this remedy have wet hands, talk too much, laugh hysterically, stutter when speaking, and are sensitive to their surroundings, like a porcelain doll. Mimulus removes their confusion. Mimulus people are less able to tolerate strong light, large amounts of food, and excessive work. If they are exposed to greater effort, they get sick, have headaches, and have problems with urination. If the pressure on them is too strong, they get sick. They have to pull it to recharge the batteries and regain energy.

Mimulus people, although timid, are very cautious and reserved and never discuss this with other people.

This type of person should get used to living with their weak constitution and, from time to time, give themselves time to rest without feeling guilty; they need to rest their nervous system.

Marina G.'s healing experience with Bach Flower Remedy:

Mimulus

Mimulus helped me overcome my fears and anxiety. His energy strengthened me and helped me face what scares me. With this remedy, I felt brave and ready to face challenges, but also to vent without remorse because of others who easily did what I needed moments of rest for.

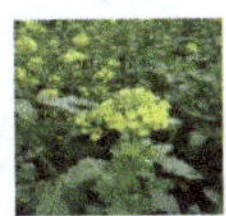

MUSTARD – Sinavis sp.

This Bach flower remedy is for a fleeting mood, for depression that comes suddenly and is of unknown origin. A person has the feeling that there is a dark cloud above him that presses him, and he wants to hide somewhere. The dark cloud disappears as it comes; it can happen in a few hours, minutes, or days. In this state, a person may have suicidal thoughts. She is melancholic, loses interest in work, etc., and has dark sadness for no apparent reason. The person has slow movements and weak motivation.

This Bach flower remedy is prescribed for:

• A grieving soul;

• Persons who are in a very bad mood;

• When he feels as if he is separated from his soul;

• Hopelessness;

• Pronounced depression;

• In teenagers whose mood changes suddenly (for example, they are very happy, and after half an hour they are sad for no apparent reason);

The vibration of the mustard essence gives a person inner security, light, stability, and cheerfulness, even in their darkest days.

Depression, 1st degree - Hornbeam,

Depression, 2nd degree - Gentian

Depression, 3rd degree - Gorse

Depression, 4th degree – Mustard

Depression, 5th degree - Sweet chestnut

Zorana M.'s healing experience with Bach Flower Remedy:

Mustard

The mustard freed me from the dark cloud of sadness and depression that oppressed me. His energy brought light and joy into my life. I feel happy and full of energy after only two months of therapy.

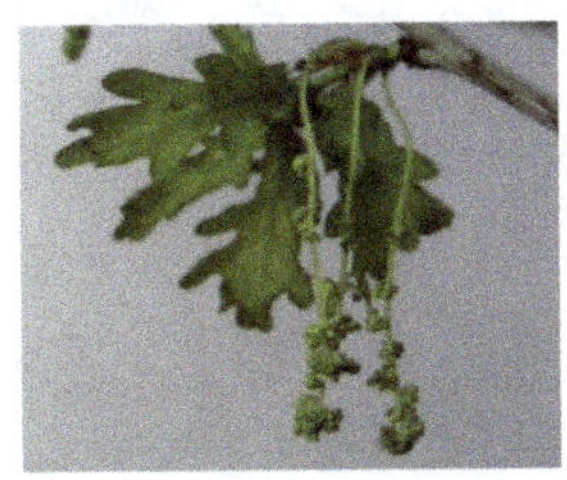

OAK – Quercus sp.

An oak remedy can be a type of person, but most often it is a remedy for a transient mood. These are people who don't pay attention to their personal needs, are overworked, don't eat, and don't sleep enough, all because of the feeling that they have to earn more, for example. They are devoted to work and forget that the meaning of life is not only in achieving success and victories; there should also be moments of relaxation and satisfaction that give strength for new victories. At the moment of overload, the body reminds us and gives us signs that we need to rest and sleep.

A person is busy with work, and this is reflected in their dreams. These are people who only think about work and are dedicated to it. But if they don't allow themselves those moments of enjoyment, then their lives become cruel and miserable. For example, mothers of the Oak type are tireless in taking care of the family; they do not allow themselves a break. They never admit that they are tired, so they end up having a nervous breakdown.

These people self-select the stress that comes with great success instead of de-stressing and balancing their personal and business lives. The characteristic of these people is that they will bite their tongue rather than seek help; they suffer if they cannot meet the expectations of the environment.

The vibration of the oak remedy is prescribed for:

• Patients on long-term sick leave, when the patient shows gradual fatigue from constant therapeutic treatments;

• Unfortunate persons who cannot perform their work due to illness;

• Dissatisfaction with oneself;

• People who have muscle spasms and sudden movements;

• Superhuman endurance;

• They do not complain to anyone;

• Those who, despite great despair, do not give up; do not lose courage;

•Even though they are faced with great problems, they look for a solution;

•If they are sick, they will try 101 remedies to get well;

Oak people are fighters who never give up; they are persistent; they fight and look for solutions when everyone else would give up. They never stop looking for the answer to everything. They do not stop hoping, even in illness, worries, accidents, problems, etc.

But despite all this courage, they have moments when they feel desperate and despondent. They suffer a lot inside, but they don't give up; they continue on their way. Endurance, determination, and persistence are their main characteristics.

They don't complain to anyone. For example, a carpenter who cuts his finger (which is a warning from his body) does not pay attention to the injury and continues to work. The next thing that happened to him was that he developed diabetes (high blood sugar).

By the way, these people are very noble; they always help others on their own initiative. The vibration of the oak remedy helps a person to relax, to pay attention to himself, to understand that he can only work if he is healthy, and to create a balance in his life. Only in this way can that person be as happy as his family because he will find time to spend with them.

A helpful thought in these situations: "From joy comes strength."

Martin J.'s healing experience with Bach Flower Remedy:

Oak

The oak remedy taught me balance and moderation. His energy reminded me that it's important to take care of yourself and not get overwhelmed by work. I feel balanced and calm. I am happy that now I have time for my family. And they are even happier.

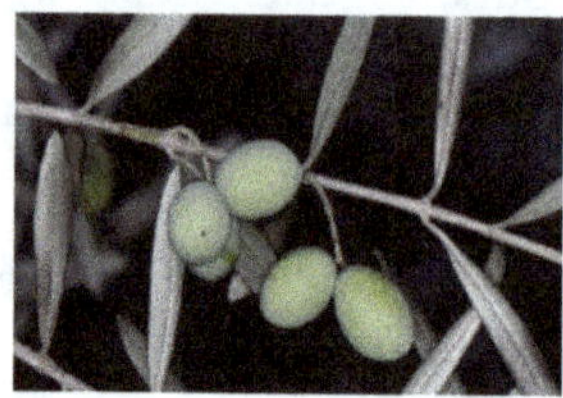

OLIVA – Olea sativa

The vibration of the Oliva remedy is always used as a mood remedy. It is associated with mental and physical exhaustion in people who study a lot (mentally exhausted) or who do heavy physical work (physical exhaustion). The vibration of this Bach flower remedy helps them relax and work more calmly and relaxedly. Very often, these people have the feeling that they are running out of strength, have a great need for sleep, and have no desire for anything. Oliva is a remedy that restores vitality and strength to people.

The vibration of this Bach flowerremedyis prescribed for:

• People who feel exhausted and tired;

• In chronic diseases as well as long-term sick leave from various diseases;

• People who do heavy physical or mental work;

• In the case of long-term insomnia;

• Severe exhaustion when both soul and body are completely tired, exhausted;

• When caring for a sick family member;

• Alcoholism;

• Various physical ailments, because it strengthens the human body and spirit;

• In cases of deep internal fatigue, when strong internal battles are being waged in the person himself, and he spends too much energy on them;

• Long-term additional work in free time;

• During recovery, or when the mind and body are not healed after some illness or some shock;

• Kidney problems;

• When a person says, This is the final straw after many years of work;

•They often know to say, " I'm ready...";

Unreasonably spending their energy on these people leads to a state of humiliation because they have to ask for help. In this state, they feel too exhausted and do not want to hear or see anyone. They are either sleeping or just sitting around doing nothing. People who fall into this state must learn to properly handle their life force and their energy.

The vibration of the olivaremedy restores peace and strength to a tired mind and body.

Marinela U.'s healing experience with Bach Flower Remedy:

Oliva

Oliva refreshed me and gave me energy when I felt exhausted and without the will to do anything in my daily life. Her energy gave me new strength and vitality. I feel energetic and renewed.

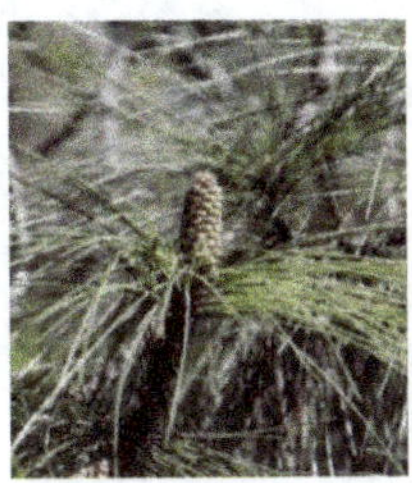

PINE - Pinus sp.

The vibration of the Bach flower remedy Pine can be a personality type or a cure for a fleeting mood. Pine is the type of person who always blames himself. They think that everything that goes wrong is their own fault. They blame themselves for events or things that are someone else's fault. They have set themselves at a much lower level than they really deserve. They often apologise.

The best example of this is when Pine, the person who enters the room, apologises first, starts the sentence with, "Sorry","Sorry for thinking's, I will never forgive myself for being so careless","I know that it's my fault that it happened" and similar statements.

The vibration of the Pine remedy is prescribed for:

• People who feel guilty about everything, despondency;

• When they keep blaming themselves for something they did in the past;

• People who deep down feel like cowards, people who work a lot and grieve a lot;

• Hypersensitive persons;

• People who judge themselves;

• Overly aware individuals;

• Humble people who constantly apologise even when there is no need for it;

• They feel sex is a sin;

• When there is no joy in one's lifestyle;

• He feels other people's mistakes as his own, with the feeling that responsibility is shared;

• children who blame themselves for their parents' divorce;

• Children who suffer because of someone else's mistake, take the blame;

• When, due to feelings of guilt, the body shows signs of exhaustion and fatigue;

• They even apologise for being sick;

• People who make sacrifices;

In general, these people are never satisfied with what they do, they always think they can do better. When their high expectations are not met, they blame themselves. Even when he achieves any kind of success, a Pina person feels inside that he didn't do something right. They have a guilt complex, with which they live in every life situation; that's why their life is gloomy. If they buy new clothes, they feel guilty. If something goes wrong at work or at home, they feel responsible, as if they are playing a game of self-pity. They set high goals for themselves and try everything to achieve them, but become depressed if they fail to live up to these high ideals.

These are people who will often help their loved ones solve a problem through patient conversation.

The positive side of using the vibration of the remedy of pine is that with it, people begin to see their positive side, their value, and the right to their own lives. By using this remedy, a person can enjoy the benefits of his own life while not taking responsibility that belongs to other people and not feeling guilty for other people's mistakes.

The vibration of the PineRemedy is that people admit their personal mistakes, accept them, do not exaggerate them, and forgive themselves.

Useful thoughts in such situations are: "I forgive myself because I haven't been forgiven for a long time" and "Every mistake is a new step towards happiness."

Mila T.'s healing experience with Bach Flower Remedy:

Pine

Pine taught me to accept my own mistakes and not judge myself all the time. His energy freed me from guilt and brought me relief. I feel liberated and blessed by my inner strength and the happiness I feel when I forgive myself for the mistake I made. Well, we are all humans and have the right to make mistakes.

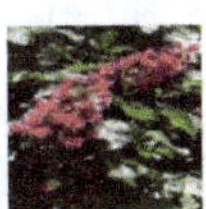

RED CHESTNUT – Aesculus X carnea

The vibration of the red chestnut flower remedy is associated with feelings of fear and concern. People don't worry about themselves, but about the well-being of their loved ones, about family, about friends, etc. A typical example of this is when a mother is waiting for her child to return from school, and she is very worried and impatient, waiting for him with the thought that something is going to happen, something bad. Another example is when the husband has to go on a business trip, and the wife thinks that something bad will happen to him on the way. These people can stand at the window and wait for hours. They are in physical spasm. They have mental and emotional spasms.

The red chestnut remedy is prescribed for:

• Fears for other people, fear of some evil;

• Too much concern for people they don't even know; and even fear for injured animals;

• They wait for the grown-up children to return home and constantly think bad things; they cannot calm down until they see that the children have returned home;

• For grandmothers who, for example, have the feeling that their heart will freeze if their grandson has to cross a busy street;

•They constantly think about the problems of others and live as if they were their own;

• They often say, "I am very worried about my father (mother), who lives alone";

• Red chestnut parents often warn their children to be very careful;

• Excessive attachment to other people;

• When babies are weaned from breastfeeding;

• Selfless care;

• When people are full of difficulties and troubles because their relationships are on an emotional, not a spiritual level;

The vibration of the red chestnut remedy allows relaxation, letting go of thoughts, and suppressing bad thoughts. With this remedy, people begin to think positively.

Robert T.'shealing experience with Bach Flower Remedy:

Red chestnut:

Red Chestnut gave me a lot of support to let go of worrying about other people. His energy brought me peace and confidence that others are capable of taking care of themselves. I feel calm and unburdened. No more constantly thinking about the problems of others and thinking that something bad will happen to my loved ones.

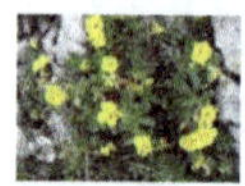

ROCK ROSE – Helianthemum sp.

The vibration of the Rock Rose remedy is a cure for fleeting moods. Rescue remedies also contain it.

It is most often prescribed for:

• Great fears and panic;

• Nightmares, fear of hearing voices, and panic attacks. This flower balances those panic attacks and brings them into a normal rhythm;

• For patients who have suffered fear of all unpleasant events, fear of surgery, and fear of illness;

• patients whose disease looks frightening;

• In cases of severe pneumonia, when the patient has a high temperature and falls unconscious;

• In severe health conditions, in life-threatening diseases (in such cases, Rock Rose should be given not only to the patient but also to the family);

• Acute states of fear that have an objective cause, when a person is very scared mentally and physically (for example, during natural disasters or incurable diseases when people are in shock or panic);

• Children who wake up at night from a nightmare;

• People who have just escaped a traffic accident;

•It is used as an additional means in the treatment of sunburn;

• With feelings of fear and panic, when people do not listen, do not see, or do not speak because of fear, when they feel as if their heart is frozen;

 • In children who often have palpitations and sweaty palms;

• In children who have taken narcotics and children who live in nervously unstable families;

• In the mother before and after childbirth;

• Nightmares and sleepwalking, screaming in sleep;

• Shock;

• Fear when a person has to face great temptations;

• With refugees;

• With people who have faced thieves;

• In any sudden, unexpected, difficult, or dangerous situation, regardless of whether it is physical, psychological, or emotional;

The vibration of this remedy stimulates the adrenal glands and balances the solar plexus. Rock Rose's condition is described as a strong shock in the abdominal region, with sweating and palpitations.

In a moment, that fear can turn into great courage. For example, when a mother saves her child from a dangerous situation or shows the bravery of a soldier, then people surpass themselves in their strength and courage.

Jane K.'s healing experience with Bach Flower Remedy:

Rock Rose

Rock Rose gave me tremendous support and help in dealing with my intense fear and panic. His energy calmed me down and gave me the inner courage to face challenges. After using this remedy, a feeling of boldness, courage, and calm prevails for me.

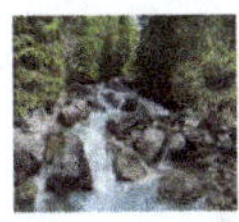

ROCK WATER – Alpine water

This is the only remedy from the group of Bach Flower Remedies that is not a flower remedy but water. Most often, it is a type of person. It is known that the largest part of our body is water, and water is the element of emotions. As a personality type, this is a strong, principled person with firm ideas and a firm way of life. They are self-disciplined, strict people who teach others by their example. If they discover something that is good for them, they stick to it without boasting. Then they teach others about such an attitude in life. They don't care about other people's opinions. If others accept their ideas, it's good for them; if they don't, it's good for them.

They pass on their example to others slowly and quietly (like water when it flows); they don't give lectures, but just as water slowly and quietly changes nature, these people change their environment. At the same time, self-reproach, spiritual rigidity, and physical stiffness appear in this type of person. They abstain from joy and the pleasures of life. Because of their ideal facade, they actually suffer a lot.

The vibration of rock water remedy is prescribed for:

• Self-love and asceticism;

• Suppression of essential physical and emotional needs;

• Strict vegetarians;

• When people meditate for hours;

• When women often have problems with their periods;

• When the body is sensitive to stress reactions;

• When people work and sacrifice everything to be strong and active;

• Inflexible people with very strong ideas in mind about religion and politics;

This type of person wants to be an example to those around them.

In this state, a person gives up many things that make everyday life pleasant and joyful because he believes that this is not right due to his strict outlook on life. Many Rock Water people ask themselves to achieve "holiness" on earth. They live in iron systems of principles and discipline of all kinds (for example, a person who practices yoga for hours, a strict economic life, etc.). Often, these theories and principles derive from old traditions that had their place in the past but not in the present.

These people are not interesting interlocutors. They are interested in politics, ecology, and many philosophical topics and recognise only their own thinking and consider it absolutely correct. Everything else that does not belong to their topics of thought does not interest them, and they do not pay attention to it. These people are not aware that they are suppressing their own human needs.

Extreme cases of rock water are very rare.

Sometimes some people have a need for this remedy because, at some point in their lives, they consciously or unconsciously suppress their life needs. They abstain from many things because of strict life principles, thereby losing the joy and beauty of life. A useful thought in situations like this: "I let things happen by themselves."

Majda H.'s healing experience with Bach Flower Remedy:

Rock water

My experience with Rock Water has been very positive. This remedy has taught me flexibility and acceptance of change. It helped me to relax and stop being too strict with myself and the environment. I feel free and relaxed about my expectations. Now I live the everyday joys of life.

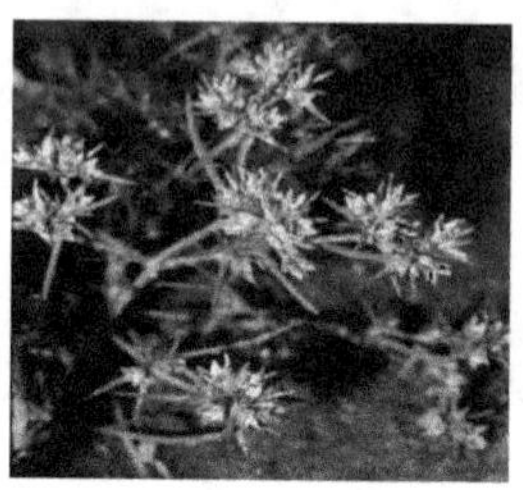

SCLERANTHUS – Scleranthus annuus

This remedy is a cure for fleeting moods and is associated with decision-making. It is most often given to people who are hesitating, unable to decide between two options. For example, when they go to the store to buy bread, they see several types of bread, and they can't decide which one to buy. As a result of indecision, they begin to suffer, become nervous, and become frustrated.

It also helps people who change their mood from sadness to joy and happiness (from extreme to extreme) in very short intervals. This often happens in children during puberty. Indecision saps their energy so that they feel exhausted. The vibration of the Scleranthus remedy helps them balance.

This remedy is prescribed for:

• Indecision;

• Lack of balance, uncertainty and anxiety;

• People who cannot decide which of two things is right;

• Because they go from extreme to extreme, they have tics and unnecessary movements;

• They don't ask anyone for advice; they often change their wardrobe;

• Objects fall out of their hands due to a lack of balance in them, they trip, jump, are clumsy, fall when climbing stairs;

• They walk unsteadily, feel dizzy;

• They refuse to surrender to the guidance of their own soul;

• Children who are restless, constantly turning around;

• Problems with the inner ear, ear infection;

• They want to find their own solution;

• Sea sickness;

• Indecisiveness, a wavering mood;

• People who waste time because of hesitation, uncertainty about what to do;

• When they are sick, their physical symptoms keep changing;

• One moment they are very nice and kind to their neighbours, and the next they can't stand them;

• They go from extreme to extreme, from excessive activity to apathy;

• One day they are too interested in an idea, and the next day they are not interested at all;

• During pregnancy;

A classic example of when the Scleranthus remedy helps is a girl who can't decide between two boyfriends, but doesn't seek advice from her parents or anyone else. She tries to make a decision on her own, even if it takes a month. These fluctuations and indecisions can cause phenomena in the body such as: hard stools and diarrhoea; increased and decreased body temperature; severe hunger and lack of appetite; high and low blood pressure; crying and laughing; and pain in one place and then another in the body.

These people lack the correct orientation of their soul, which gives strength, measure, and direction. They have an inner imbalance; they can't concentrate; they jump from topic to topic in conversation; and because of this inner vacillation, they miss many good opportunities in life and in business.

They often say, "My mind is like a restless sea" or "My mind is divided." The vibration of this remedy helps people become decisive and make immediate decisions with precise accuracy. A useful thought in such situations is, "I choose the golden path by the golden mean."

Martin D.'s healing experience with Bach Flower Remedy:

Scleranthus

Scleranthus was a great support and helped in making decisions. His energy cleared my mind and helped me focus on what was important. I feel strong and confident in my decisions. No more indecision.

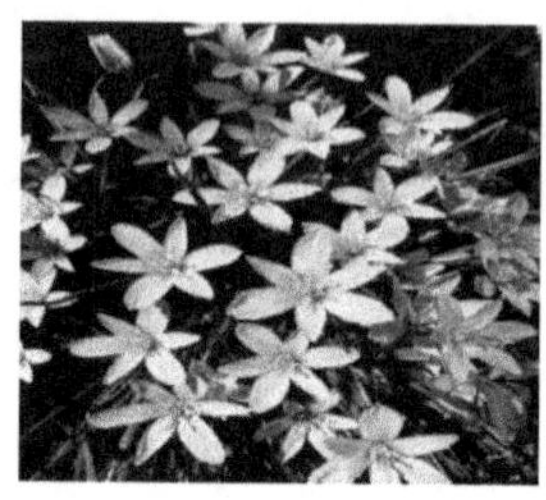

STAR OF BETHLEHEM – Ornithogalum umbellatum

The vibration of this remedy is used in states of shock, whether it is a sudden situation in the moment or a childhood shock. This flower releases emotions from the past, such as feelings of sadness, deep mourning, etc. The Star of Bethlehem is the most important flower in the combination of drops for first aid (rescue remedy), which unifies the vibrational action of the other flowers.

The term shock refers to any excessively strong energy action that the human body cannot neutralise, and the body reacts by disrupting the balance. At some point in life, every person experiences emotional traumas that they cannot cope with. Some of them are immediately reflected on the physical level. Any shock to the body can lead to the onset of arthritis. Many psychosomatic diseases arise as a result of unresolved energy traumas, to which each person reacts differently depending on which organ in the body is weaker.

The Star of Bethlehem remedy rarely appears as a trait in people's characters. In this state, people are very nice and quiet when they speak; their voice becomes quieter at the end of the sentence, and they move slowly.

The vibration of the Star of Bethlehem remedy is prescribed for:

• Conditions that are the result of a survived shock, regardless of whether it is psychological, physical, or mental, and regardless of whether it happened today, the day before, or many years ago;

• People inclined towards the magical and mystical;

• When a person closes in on himself;

• When losing a loved one after a serious accident;

• Severe, deep sadness, shock, and bad news;

• A remedy for people who are in great distress, suffering, and exhaustion due to accidents and conditions that cause severe and deep grief;

• People who do not accept comfort;

• The consequences of shock that affect a person physically and mentally;

• Loss of a loved one;

• Inner spiritual stiffness;

• Postpartum trauma;

• Speaking quietly;

• Attempted poisoning;

• For children after the divorce of their parents, it is given together with Walnut (for adaptation to the new situation);

• Psychosomatic diseases; feeling of tension in the throat; nervous disorders when swallowing;

•Loss of hearing and sight; problems with walking;

• In women with heavy menstrual bleeding;

• In people who are sad and paralysed after experiencing disappointments (unpleasant experiences that remain in consciousness for a long, long time);

• For newborns, this remedy is recommended together with the walnut remedy due to the shock at birth and adaptation to new living conditions (drops can also be put in the baby's bath water);

The vibrationof the Star of Bethlehem remedy dissolves the sediment; it is like a catalyst for all obstacles - a comforter and a means to alleviate grief. After using this remedy, a person becomes more active, his mental strength increases, and he gains energy. This remedy is called a soul comforter and pain reliever.

A useful suggestive thought in this state is: "I release blocked energies" and "My head is clear and clear."

Robert E.'s healing experience with Bach Flower Remedy:

Star of Bethlehem

The Star of Bethlehem helped me overcome emotional trauma and the loss of my beloved wife. His energy brought me comfort and relief and helped me in the process of mental and physical healing. Now I feel calm and emotionally strong.

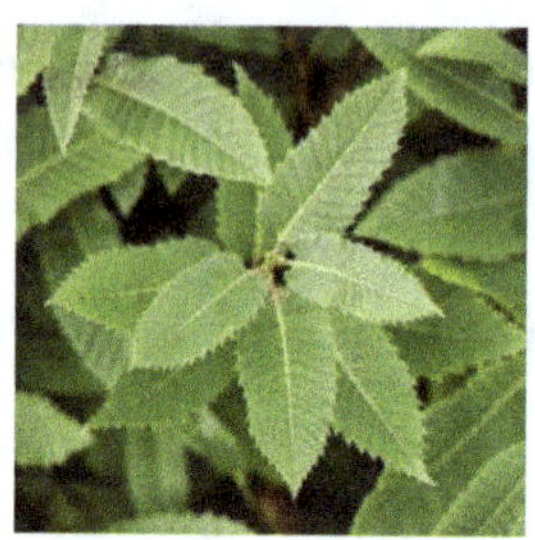

SWEET CHESTNUT – Castanea sativa

The vibration of the sweet chestnut remedy is used for great fears and the deepest depression when people feel that there is no light at the end of the tunnel. A person has the feeling that this is the end of his life. Often, these people think about suicide. It is a very difficult state of mind and soul.

This Bach flower remedy is prescribed for:

• People who say that there is no way out for them, no help, and no hope to stay alive;

• Despair, hopelessness, and inner pain;

• Unbearable mental suffering;

• People who have a complete emptiness inside;

• Brave people who face life's trials on their own and control the situation in which only disappointment and emptiness remain. This suffering can be physical or psychological;

• A future in complete darkness, complete loneliness, and intense mental suffering;

• People who have hit rock bottom. A very negative state of mind;

• When a person is alone against everyone,the person feels as if they are hanging in the air;

• An empty, almost hopeless present. The moment of truth, the dark night of the soul transformation phase;

• For people who experience mental pain and despair for a shorter or longer period of time, for whom all hope has disappeared;

• Deep despair when a person no longer knows what to do;

• He feels that he has reached the ultimate limits of endurance;

• Severe depression when there is no hope;

• They hide their feelings and problems from others around them;

In this state, a person feels completely helpless and unprotected, like a chicken that has fallen out of the nest. They are convinced that there is no hope for them because they are suffering too much.

The vibration of the sweet chestnut remedy opens up new possibilities for a person and helps to see the bright side. He feels that life is worth living and gets the courage to move on in life. A person with this Bach flower remedy finds himself.

A thought that helps in this situation is: "When the trouble is the hardest, God's help is the closest."

Sonja G.'s healing experience with Bach Flower Remedy:

Sweet chestnut

Sweet Chestnut has provided me with support and help at times when I have faced deep anxiety, despair, and the feeling that this is the end of me. There is no more hope for me. His energy brought me hope and a new perspective. Now I am full of energy, faith, and enthusiasm for new achievements in life.

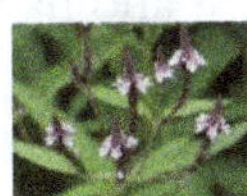

VERVAIN – Verbena officinalis

The flower vibration of the Vervain remedy can be a personality type or used for mood. Vervain people have enormous enthusiasm, ideas, and methods to fight for. They act impatiently and try to spread their idea at any cost, reach as many people as possible, and realise it in the shortest possible time. This type of person gives lectures all the time. They want to have followers who will support their methods. They are often annoying to the environment because, for example, they force people to attend various workshops. And if their friends don't accept, then they are very angry. It can also be a person who strongly wants to help someone.

A Vervain person is always in a hurry; he doesn't have time to finish everything he wants. Their lives are full of obligations. They remind me of the famous sentence, "What is this life worth if we don't have time to stop for a moment and enjoy its beauty?". They don't have time all the time, and because of that, they miss many beauties in life and nature around them. They have a lot of mental energy that they need to balance. They are too enthusiastic, they exert themselves too much, and they do everything with tension.

These people can fall into a state of stress due to too much ambition and enthusiasm (they take on many obligations). Because they are great enthusiasts, they think a lot at night and have too many impressions, so they can't sleep. They feel nervous energy moving through their muscles. If you hold these people's hands, you will be able to feel their tension. Due to this condition, they often suffer from rheumatic pain and stiffness, and all this is due to their constant tense state.

Bach flower remedy Vervain is prescribed for:

• Individuals who are brave and continue to fight even in a state of illness;

• People who do more harm than good;

• Terrible muscle tension;

• Sensitive to injustice, whether at home or at a friend's house;

• People who live very fast and burn out quickly like a match;

• When people get tired too quickly, they live tensely, and this exhausts them; they feel sick and broken;

• When their mind wanders, strong, great rapture;

• Fanatic type of person;

•A reformer trying to change the world has fixed ideas that they are sure are correct;

•Internal tension, inability to relax;

• For people whose inner will and conviction have led them to live in a state of constant tension and who have imposed it on themselves;

• For people who are convinced that they are right and want to convince others that they are right about some idea. They simply press on them with their energy and tyre them out;

• They are irritable if things do not go as they imagined;

• They don't allow themselves a minute of rest;

• Perfectionists who are not satisfied with anything;

• They work continuously, regardless of their borders;

• They do not use their own energy properly;

Children of this type are very active, and at night, it is very difficult to convince them to go to sleep.

Often, this type of person gets sick, for example, from the flu, because they draw energy from the body's protective forces (immunity). Some people are so troubled inside that they cannot afford physical rest. These are people who don't know how to keep their mouths shut and are ready to go behind bars for their ideals.

The vibration of the Vervain essence helps these people see that there are many ways out of the world's problems and that everyone can find their own way of life. This Bach flower remedy helps them to accept that there are other ways of thinking besides their own. It teaches them to have a broader view of the world. Stick to your opinion and ideas, but also recognise the right of others to their opinion.

Jasna C.'s healing experience with Bach Flower Remedy:

Vervain

Vervain taught me balance and moderation in my attitudes and beliefs. His energy soothed me and brought me inner peace. I felt balanced and freely expressed my opinion. At the same time, I respected the opinions of the people around me.

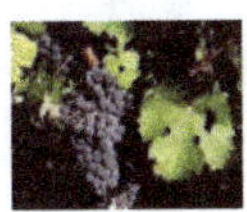

VINE – Vitis vinifera

Vine -type people are dominant, have strong opinions, and always want to be right. They often say, "You will not tell me; you will do as I tell you". They can't stand other people's opinions and want theirs to be accepted. They terrorise everyone in the family because they want everything to be as they say. They lack tolerance. Vine people are good leaders and teachers.

When they learn what tolerance is, they will be firm in their views, but they will also be understanding, and they will be gentle and able to accept other people's opinions. They are too confident in their success and abilities. These people are very capable, strong-willed, irritable, self-confident, and have a desire to dominate and command. In the role of the patient, they control the doctor and the nurse because they are calm, composed, and cruel because they feel they know best.

The vibration of the Vine remedyis prescribed for:

• Ambitious people who love power and authority;

• Excessive ambitions and inflexibility;

• They act without thinking;

• Rigid and unyielding, they set rules and have no compassion for others;

• They can behave tyrannically towards the environment;

• They have a habit of giving orders;

• Individuals who thrive, unscrupulous;

• In sudden, difficult circumstances;

• With migraines and high blood pressure due to tension;

• People who want to do good to others, whether they like it or not;

• People who think they know everything better than others and that everyone should do as they say;

• Authority, greed for power;

• They have no respect for the peculiarities of other people;

• They are unsurpassed when it comes to strength, will, and poise;

• They are merciless, cruel;

• They find a way out of every crisis;

• People who do evil, thieves, criminals;

• A domestic tyrant and dictator who does not want to argue because he is always right;

Children of this type brutally mistreat children in their class.

In the final stage, these people are very authoritative, eager for power, and have no respect for the individuality of their fellow human beings. Vine energy represents a very strong form of energy, which gives these people the quality of leaders who set high expectations for themselves. But they actually use that power to satisfy their limited egoistic goals. These people are unsurpassed in strength of will and spirit and always hold the reins in their hands. I cannot understand the attitude of other people and convince them to do as they say and that it is for their own good.

Many evildoers and tyrants in world history, from the time of Dionysus to Neron, were vine types.

In the state of vine, a person completely loses judgement about others and acts extremely subjective and self-confident. An example of this is a father who says, "I have to hold my son tight," not taking into account that the son feels fear for him instead of affection. Or a teacher who says, "Don't think, but do what I tell you."

The state of Vine can cause various physical ailments, which are an expression of strong inner tension, high pressure, various types of neuroses, physical pain, etc. Vine people are very capable, extremely self-confident, and have great ego strength. He is a domestic tyrant and dictator who does not talk because he is always right.

A useful suggestive thought in this situation is: "To rule is to serve." "I understand and respect the uniqueness of each person."

Sara S.'s healing experience with Bach Flower Remedy:

Vine

Vine taught me to be a leader, to give orders, but also to be flexible in my leadership. The energy of this essence gave me a sense of respect and understanding for the needs of others. I felt inspired and happy because others around me felt beautiful and respected and still listened to my views.

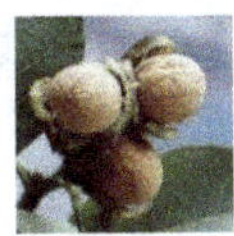

WALNUT – Juglans regia

This remedy can be a personality type, but it is also used for fleeting moods. The vibration of this Bach flower remedy is about protection. It is a cure for all people who cannot adapt to any change, whether it is a change of residence, change of job, menopause, new teacher, retirement, going to another school - in fact, any change. It is successfully given to the newborn after birth because it is a time of change, as well as to the mother during pregnancy. It has great success with teenagers because big changes happen during puberty.

The vibration of the walnut remedy is prescribed for:

• Climax in women and men;

• In old patients before death, because this is also a change when great uncertainty is felt;

• It helps to break the old way of thinking and start a new life;

•The remedy breaks old addictions;

•A remedy for those who want to change but simply cannot get rid of old habits and thoughts;

• Uncertainty in a period of change; becoming more confident in one's attitudes and not being influenced by the opinions and views of the environment;

• For people who allow others to change their minds in their decisions (example for work, travel, etc.);

• In babies, while their teeth are growing;

• When making important decisions in life;

• When getting married, changing jobs;

• When converting to another religion;

• When entering into a partnership, changing occupations;

• When the time for retirement approaches;

• When voluntarily going to a nursing home;

• In the event of a stroke or any other life-changing illness;

• When a person starts working in an environment that he cannot stand;

• During psychotherapy;

• In the case of divorce;

• To retain energy in homoeopathic treatment;

• Addiction support;

• Final stage of the disease;

• Change of apartment or move abroad (helps in adapting a person to a new environment);

Increasing changes lead to significant stress and increased inner uncertainty. A man in the state of Walnut has clear goals in life and knows what he wants, but in those difficult moments, he cannot remain consistent with himself.

The vibration of the walnut remedy always helps us to be more relaxed and harmonious. This remedy gives permanence. It helps a person move forward towards the realisation of his tasks and goals in his own life, regardless of the inner state and opinion of other people.

Useful suggestive thoughts in the Walnut state: "I follow my inner impulses", "I am resilient".

Marjan C.'shealing experience with Bach Flower Remedy:

Walnut

Walnut supported me in the process of change and adaptation. His energy gave me strength and self-confidence and helped me protect myself from environmental influences. I felt safe and protected as I walked the path of change. I followed my dream.

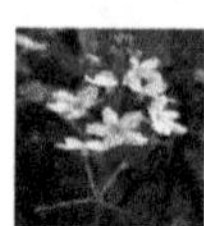

WATER VIOLET – Hottonia palustris

In the Water Violet state, people are very quiet, have a lot of self-confidence, know their purpose in life, and stand firmly on the ground with their attitudes. The people around them feel inferior (lower than them). But it only looks that way because people of the Water Violet type only look proud, but in reality they are not. In the eyes of others, they seem unattainable. They really like to help people around them, but they are not forced to do so. They quietly perform their duties. If someone asks them for help, they will be happy to help.

They are talented, wise, and extremely good at dealing with special or difficult situations. As people, they are calm and dignified; they like to work alone; and they carry their deep sorrows and problems in silence. They do not interfere in other people's business, which is why they do not accept other people's help even when they are sick. They want to deal with their own problems. All of this leads them to block energy, which eventually leads to back and neck problems.

The vibration of the Bach flower remedy Water violet is prescribed for:

• Pride, reserve, arrogance, and proud isolation;

• People who want to be alone in health and illness;

• Calm people who speak in a low tone and do not respect the opinions of others around them;

• They do not show their feelings and are withdrawn into themselves;

• They go their own way and do not bother others;

• People who choose their own path and cannot be easily influenced;

• Individuals who radiate wisdom. As managers, they are highly respected because they perform their work very conscientiously and with tact and composure. They never force employees to do something they don't want to do, unlike the Vine guy, who does just that;

The environment loves Water Violet people too much, but they, on the contrary, like to be alone. If they overdo it in isolation, they begin to suffer. They want to have friends, hang out, but still be alone. When they realise that they are completely alone, they become sad because there is no one around them. Then these individuals need the vibration of the water violet flower. This condition can lead to health issues.

Often, when teachers and healers want to completely isolate themselves from the world, this remedy is recommended to them. The positive effect of the Water Violet vibration is that a person begins to protect and take care of friendships, visit friends, invite guests, etc.Simply create a balance in their lives.

Suggestive thought in this state: "I need friends, and they need me."

Marijana B.'s healing experience with Bach Flower Remedy:

Water Violet

Water Violet taught me how to be more open to other people. His energy encouraged me to be approachable and compassionate. I felt connected and fulfilled as I shared my energy with others around me.

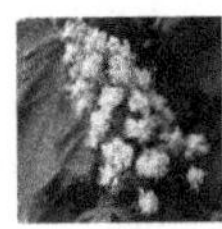

WHITE CHESTNUT – Aesculus hippocastanum

The vibration of the White Chestnut remedy can be a personality type, but it is also used for a transient mood. This is a remedy for persistent worrying thoughts and mental arguments within yourself. The result is insufficient sleep, and the person wakes up tired as if he had worked all night. Their body is tired. This mental confusion can also happen during the day when our thoughts do not give us peace.

It helps when people are too worried and can't sleep at night. Or they wake up at night and have a dialogue with themselves; they can't stop their thoughts; they lie down and can't fall asleep. Such unwanted thoughts can lead to headaches, especially in the front of the head in the eye area.

The vibration of the white chestnut remedy is prescribed for:

• Dark thoughts that I cannot get out of my head (people have difficulty falling asleep or wake up very early);

• People who feel like their mind is like a record that keeps spinning and never stops;

• Unwanted thoughts that keep coming back and interfere with work or pleasures at a given moment;

• They have conversations and dialogues with themselves; their thoughts pile on top of each other;

• They often say, "My thoughts don't stop moving and talking";

• Loss of concentration;

This type of person feels internally burdened by thoughts that are constantly running through their head, and they cannot get rid of them. Their inner tension can be expressed by grinding their teeth during sleep and by tension in their eyes and forehead.

The vibration of the white chestnut remedy stabilises a person and helps him find a solution to his thoughts and the right solution to the problems that bother him. It brings balance and calming thoughts.

Suggestive thoughts in this state: "I am filled with calm", "Everything is happening in order".

Jasna I.'shealing experience with Bach Flower Remedy:

White chestnut

The white chestnut freed me from the constant thoughts and worries that were running through my head. His energy soothed me and brought me inner peace. Now I feel calm and focused on the present moment.

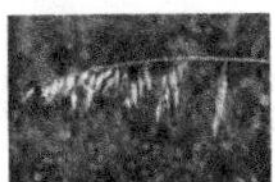

WILD OAT – Avena fatua

This Bach flower remedy is most often used for a passing mood, but it can also be a personality type. These are people who have the ambition to do something important in their lives. They want to live very intensely, but they cannot decide what to do. They become dissatisfied and desperate. They waste a lot of time on this indecision.

This is the remedy associated with making important decisions in life. People have the feeling that they are at a crossroads and do not know which direction to choose. An example of this is the choice of profession among students when choosing a school, college, etc. The vibration of this flower remedy helps them make a decision.

The vibration of wild oat remedy is prescribed for:

• Midlife crisis;

• People who are amateurs in many things;

• Sexual problems;

• Overeating;

• People who do not give up but continue with their goal;

• People who spend their energy;

• When a person does some work but thinks that it is not for him and, at the same time, does not know what else to do. They become insecure and hesitant to leave their old job and start a new one;

• Selfish and self-absorbed;

• Children who are members of a criminal family;

• Uncertainty, despondency, and difficulty in finding the right path in life;

• Feeling of inner emptiness;

• The eternal bachelor who never reaches the finish line;

• They have many ideas, representations, and desires;

• They dissipate their energy in many directions instead of focusing it on one goal under their own guidance;

Wild oat people are very talented, but the key word for them is indecision and dissatisfaction. They change many professions. The work they initially did with great desire and joy now becomes boring and uninteresting, like the colleagues they work with. Therefore, they destroy what they have achieved in order to start a new job that they think will bring them a sense of greater satisfaction.

Often, wild oats type peoplecan be very talented children who don't need to work hard to achieve what they want. They easily achieve what they imagine. The vibration of the wild oat remedy allows people to have clear ideas and the determination to make the right decision. Very often, this remedy is used when all others fail.

Daniel O.'s healing experience with Bach Flower Remedy:

Wild oat

Wild oats helped me find purpose and direction in my life. His energy directed me to what fulfils me and brought clarity to my goals. I made the decision easily. I felt inspired and strong in my search for the true purpose of my life.

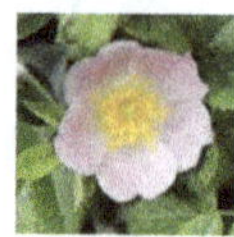

WILD ROSE – Rosa canina

The vibration of this Bach flower remedy can be a personality type or can be used as a remedy for a current mood. This type of person is apathetic and has no motivation in life. When they are sick, they surrender to the disease. People who have come to terms with their fate, be it their daily work, illness, or unhappy life. They don't complain, but they don't do anything to help themselves or get out of that situation.

These are people without joy in themselves. It is a period of stagnation in life when a person does not progress in a given situation or in life in general. This condition can also occur due to the influence of the environment when a person does not have the strength and motivation to change something.

A wild rose flower remedy is prescribed for:

• Despondency, apathy, and people who surrender to life without motivation;

• They do not have their own initiative;

• People who only vegetate;

• Mentally paralysed;

• People without interest in life who hope for nothing and do nothing to change their lives for the better;

• Feeling of sadness, indifference, and inner emptiness;

• They look like wilting flowers;

• Boring and demanding partners because they are hard on the environment;

These people live life without initiative.That is, they take as much as life gives them. They say, "Such is fate". They overcame depression, surrendered, and came to terms with that condition. They don't believe that anything can change. They often say, "It's a family trait" or "Everything is over for me".

A helpful suggestive thought for this state is: "I feel that my life is becoming happier, more interesting, and more active".

Kole V.'shealing experience with Bach Flower Remedy:

Wild rose

Wild roses encouraged me to move and to accept that life can be filled with experiences and joys. His energy woke me up and gave me new motivation. I felt alive and happy, enjoying every moment the day had to offer.

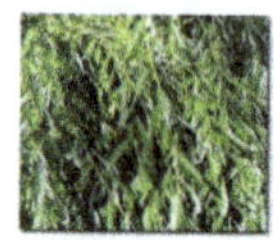

WILLOW – Salix sp.

The vibration of Bach flower remedies Willow can be a personality type, but it is often given for a fleeting mood. It is prescribed for people who, when they are dissatisfied with life, are offended, angry, or bitter, always blame others for their bad situation, and never blame themselves. They never apologize. They often say, "God is to blame; there is no God, if there was one, he would help me", "I am miserable", or "What did I do to deserve this?".

These individuals feel that they did not deserve such an evil fate and that they were wronged. They see themselves as victims and envy others for their good health, happiness, and success.

The vibration of Willow remedyis prescribed and helps for:

• People who cannot understand that their negative attitude is responsible for their fate;

•When they mourn their fate and expect condolences from their loved ones;

• They do not accept responsibility for their lives;

• They publicly express their disappointments and resentment;

• They feel that they are victims;

• Mood and resentment towards life;

• They block the guidance of their own selves;

• They are always in a dark mood;

• Resentful of life, they make vicious remarks and spoil the mood of the people around them;

• They blame someone else for their failure, even jokingly;

• Difficulty accepting misfortune;

• They feel that life treats them badly;

• Half-heartedly admits feeling better during recovery (they say, "I may look good, but you don't know how I feel");

• They say," Poor me";

• Bitterness;

• Everyone is wrong, only he is right;

• Eternal patients who go from doctor to doctor for an opinion;

These are people who spoil the good mood in society, sow a bad mood, always complain about life, and do not appreciate the joy that life brings. Most often, this condition occurs in people who have passed middle age and begin to grumble that they have achieved little of their ideals and desires (an example is a manager who has to cede his workplace to a subordinate).

They can carry resentment towards a person in their hearts for years without showing it publicly. At the same time, they may have occasional rheumatic complaints. They are like a volcano that always smokes but never erupts. In the Willow state, a person feels like a victim. This is how he finds justification for himself - that he does not bear responsibility for his anger.

They constantly grumble, find fault, and cannot understand how others around them can be so carefree. This condition can become chronic, which can have a destructive effect on the person and the environment. Like a rotten apple that destroys the other apples around it.

The vibration of the Willow remedy helps a person understand and accept that only he is responsible for his life. To look and analyse themselves before blaming someone. It gives courage, energy, and activity to move through life.

Petra R.'s healing experience with Bach Flower Remedy:

Willow

Willow taught me to let go of negative emotions like anger or rage. His energy freed me from the burden and brought me inner peace. I felt free and freed from negativity. I stopped blaming others for the events in my life.

ABOUT THE AUTHOR

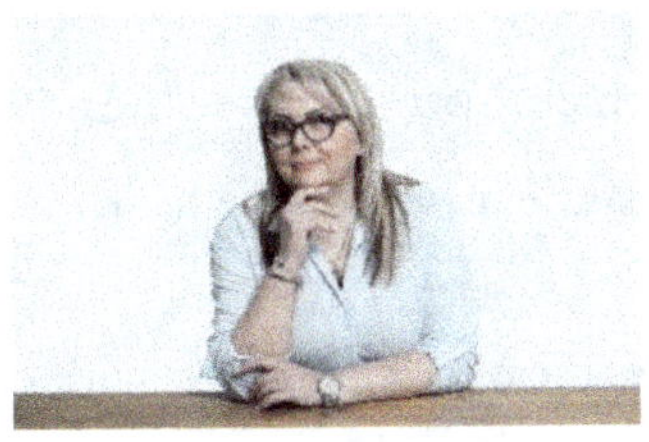

I am Zaklina Zic, a successful businesswoman, mother, daughter, best friend, and happy grandmother. I worked as a nurse in Skopje for 30 years. I graduated in business management in London and in Healing with homoeopathy and Bach flower therapy. I am also a certified life coach and mentor.

Today I work as a life coach and mentor, a holistic practitioner of homoeopathy, and a Bach flower remedy.

Why do I believe in the power of natural medicine?

I believe because I have walked that path of change and healing. Using alternative medicine - homoeopathy and Bach flower remedies - helped me regain my lost health and build strong self-confidence. I used them 20 years ago, and I still use them today when I need them.

I was full of fears and indecisiveness, like you, for a long time. I always asked myself first: what other people will say, what if they don't accept my decisions, what if I lose these people from my life, and many more questions. I spent hours and days in thoughts that produced no results. I was stuck in that endless cycle, always repeating the same actions, habits, and beliefs. I couldn't achieve results that would make me happy, healthy, and full of energy and love for myself and all the people around me.

Today, I live a life in which I primarily feel healthy, satisfied, and happy. Today, I am the absolute creator of my own life.

That is why today I am dedicated to working with clients whom I help with Bach flower therapy and homoeopathy to bring their health and lives into balance. Today, I support my clients in solving life situations, their personal development, and achieving goals for a healthy and happy life, because I am sure that anyone who decides to succeed and believes in himself can achieve it.